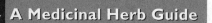

P9-DUF-669

# Herbs for Hepatitis C and the Liver

Stephen Harrod Buhner

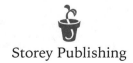

Storey Publishing

*The mission of Storey Publishing is to serve our customers
by publishing practical information that encourages
personal independence in harmony with the environment.*

Edited by Deborah Balmuth
Cover design by Meredith Maker
Cover art production and text design by Betty Kodela
Text production by Jennifer Jepson Smith
Illustrations on pages 26, 29, 42, 47, 56, 62, and 74 by Alison Kolesar;
  other illustrations by Sarah Brill, Beverly Duncan, and Mallory Lake
Indexed by Peggy Holloway
Technical review by Paul Bergner

Printed in the United States by Versa Press
20  19  18  17  16  15  14  13  12  11  10  9

### Library of Congress Cataloging-in-Publication Data

Buhner, Stephen Harrod.
    Herbs for hepatitis C and the liver / Stephen Harrod Buhner.
        p. cm. — (A Storey medicinal herb guide)
    Includes index.
    ISBN-13: 978-1-58017-255-4 (pbk.)
    ISBN-10: 1-58017-255-5 (pbk.)
    1. Hepatitis C — Alternative treatment.    2. Herbs — Therapeutic use.
3. Liver — Diseases — Alternative treatment.    4. Hepatitis C — Diet
therapy. 5. Liver — Diseases — Diet therapy. I. Title. II. Medicinal herb guide.
RC848.H425 B847 2000
616.3'62306 — dc21                                                    00-034454

# CONTENTS

1 Hepatitis C: The Silent Epidemic . . . . . . . . . . . . . . . . . . . .1

2 Hepatitis C, the Liver, and the Immune System . . . . . .14

3 Botanical Medicines for Hepatitis C and the Liver . . . .24

4 Botanical Support for the Immune System . . . . . . . . . .55

5 Nutritional Supplements for Hepatitis C . . . . . . . . . . .76

6 Changing Your Diet: Giving Your Liver a Break . . . . . .83

7 The Complete HCV Protocol . . . . . . . . . . . . . . . . . . . .96

**Epilogue:** Aggressive Symbionts: The Specter
of Emerging Viruses . . . . . . . . . . . . . . . . . . . . . . . . . . .102

**Appendix 1:** Tests for Hepatitis C and
What They Mean . . . . . . . . . . . . . . . . . . . . . . . . . . . . . .111

**Appendix 2:** Making and Using Herbal
Medicines for Hepatitis and the Liver . . . . . . . . . . . . . .113

Resources . . . . . . . . . . . . . . . . . . . . . . . . . . . . . . . . . . . .119

Suggested Reading . . . . . . . . . . . . . . . . . . . . . . . . . . . . .120

Glossary . . . . . . . . . . . . . . . . . . . . . . . . . . . . . . . . . . . . .121

Selected Bibliography . . . . . . . . . . . . . . . . . . . . . . . . . . .124

Index . . . . . . . . . . . . . . . . . . . . . . . . . . . . . . . . . . . . . . . .147

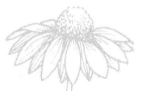

# DEDICATION

To my sister, Cathy Buhner Guido;
to Donald Yance, Matthew Dolan,
and Frank Ryan for their work;
and to the hepatitis C and Epstein-Barr viruses,
which have taught me more than books
ever could about the intelligence
of the viral world.

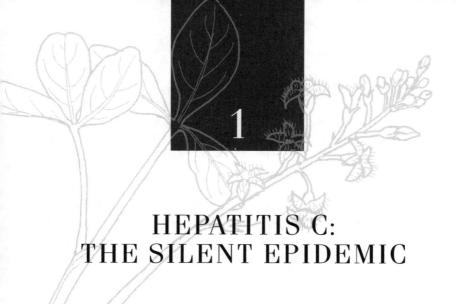

# HEPATITIS C:
# THE SILENT EPIDEMIC

It is silent, hidden, without symptoms for years, found by accident. Five hundred million people on Earth have it. It is hepatitis C virus (HCV) infection.

In the industrialized world, it's usually discovered like this: Someone goes to the doctor for a checkup, complaining of feeling tired, or he applies for insurance coverage. A routine blood test is conducted. "I am sorry," the physician or insurance company says, "you have tested positive for hepatitis C." The insurance company may deny coverage and the physician, depending on her training, will usually do one of two things.

If the physician has seen some of the problems that advanced HCV infection can cause, the information she will share with her patient is often frightening and not very encouraging. She will suggest interferon therapy if the liver enzyme levels are not too high and if the patient doesn't have cirrhosis. If the physician knows little about the disease, he will often dismiss it as "nothing much." Often the patient finds, years later, as symptoms become increasingly uncomfortable, that there is something to worry about after all.

Hepatitis C is in fact a serious disease, and it is here to stay. As Robert Goldstein of Baylor University Medical Center warns, "[Hepatitis C] is going to make the AIDS epidemic look pale."

# INFECTION AND DISEASE FROM HCV

In most cases, hepatitis C is blood-borne, and the virus presumably needs to enter the body through contaminated blood in a cut or injection. Unlike HIV, HCV is not fragile. No one knows how long it can survive in microscopic traces of dried blood; after 3 months, it is still active and infectious. Fortunately, person-to-person infection, even through sex, is extremely rare (only about 2 percent of infections are caused this way). More worrisome is that for 10 to 20 percent of people with the disease, the route of infection cannot be determined. New research indicates that HCV can live and reproduce in mosquitos (like a number of viral relatives of HCV, such the as yellow fever virus). This raises the very real possibility that HCV is transmitted through mosquito bites.

## Incubation Period

The incubation period of HCV before symptoms occur can be as long as 50 years, although the average is 15 to 25 years. If the disease goes untreated, the prognosis can be grim. Seventy percent of infected people will develop some kind of chronic liver disease, 15 percent will have cirrhosis of the liver, and 5 percent will die. Only about 10 to 15 percent seem to remain unaffected by the disease. HCV infection is now the number one cause of liver transplantation in the United States.

## PRIMARY SYMPTOMS OF HEPATITIS C

The primary symptoms of hepatitis C may include nonspecific consistent fatigue, malaise, confusion and short-term memory problems, mood swings, increased allergies, skin eruptions and itching, fluid retention in the lower extremities, consistent mild flulike symptoms, intolerance to alcohol, intolerance to fat, and depression. Pain in the liver sometimes occurs. Jaundice is rare, although common problems include bile duct damage, lymphoid aggregates, and steatosis.

It is estimated that 2 percent of the population of the industrialized world is infected: this includes some 5 to 6 million people in the United States and about 1.2 million people in the United Kingdom. The incidence of infection in other parts of the world is much higher — up to

10 percent of people in China, India, and Africa. Of the 5 to 6 million infected people in the United States, only 1 million have been diagnosed. Every year, 150,000 to 170,000 new cases are found, and 8000 to 10,000 people die. The number of deaths is expected to triple by 2007. HCV infection is the most common cause of liver disease, cirrhosis, and liver cancer in the western world.

## Conventional Treatment

Conventional medical treatment for hepatitis C focuses on the use of interferon (an immune stimulant) and ribavirin (an antiviral drug). This treatment can be quite expensive, sometimes has severe side effects, and is only partly effective. Only about half of the people with hepatitis C fit the treatment profile and will be given interferon. Of those, about half will show viral clearance after a year of treatment. In this group, half will show a resurgence of the virus after discontinuing interferon therapy. The effectiveness rate is about 15 percent. If interferon is combined with ribavirin, these rates double for patients who fit the treatment profile, up to about 35 percent effectiveness. Ribavirin alone (600 mg orally twice daily) for 12 months reduces alanine aminotransferase levels (although these levels rise again after treatment ceases) but does not affect viral levels in the blood. Researchers comment that "ribavirin clearly has no antiviral effect" on HCV. However, interferon plus ribavirin seems to have a synergistic effect. Interferon or interferon plus ribavirin is usually indicated for patients with low liver enzyme levels and no signs of cirrhosis.

The most common side effect of interferon (for about 80 percent of patients) is similar to a moderate case of the flu — for the whole year of treatment. Diarrhea and depression can also occur. The primary side effect of ribavirin is hemolysis (destruction of red blood cells). The treatment is quite expensive for patients without insurance, up to $10,000 or more per year. And, again, it is effective only for about one-third of those treated. Furthermore, both interferon and ribavirin are designed only to deal with the presence of the virus; they do nothing to heal damage to the liver or other systemic effects of the disease.

For most of the people in the world, for those without insurance, those who are not candidates for interferon–ribavirin therapy, and those in whom the therapy fails, no other medical options are available.

## THE HEPATITIS C VIRUS

HCV is a remarkable virus. (I know, I have it.) It is one of the tiniest known. In comparison, the smallpox virus is one of the largest; it can actually be seen through a microscope, although even with the best lenses it is only a tiny speck.

By a not-too-far stretch of the imagination, smallpox looks like a knobby, squarish brick. (Some researchers actually call the virus that.) And if you took three million smallpox viruses and laid them down like brick pavers for a patio floor, they would just about cover the period at the end of this sentence. So, if a smallpox brick were the size of a real brick, then a cold virus would be a blueberry sitting on top of it. HCV is

## THE HEPATITIS A VIRUS

Hepatitis A has long been recognized as a specific disease, although the virus itself was not isolated until 1973. The hepatitis A virus (HAV) is transmitted from peoples' feces into food or water or shellfish and from there to other people. Hepatitis A is usually a short-term, self-resolved illness accompanied by jaundice, diarrhea, vomiting, and lethargy. It is considered dangerous for young infants, the elderly, and people with hepatitis C. It is most common in nonindustrial countries, although outbreaks from contaminated restaurant food are not all that uncommon in the United States and Europe.

Evidence suggests that people with chronic hepatitis C who also contract hepatitis A are at increased risk for fulminant liver failure (which almost invariably results in death). A fairly recent study following 432 HCV-infected patients noted that during the 7 years of the study, 17 contracted HAV. Of those 17, 7 developed fulminant liver failure, and all but 1 of those 7 died. Other studies do not show this same high rate, but they still link an increased liver failure rate with combined HCV and HAV infection. Many physicians strongly suggest that patients with chronic hepatitis C receive HAV vaccination, especially if they are traveling in developing countries. Because shellfish filter the water in lakes, rivers, and oceans, they can build up high levels of HAV in their bodies. People with hepatitis C should avoid all shellfish.

one-third the size of that blueberry, about 30 to 35 nanometers (thousands of a millionth of a meter). This incredibly small size has made HCV very hard to study. Only now is it coming to be understood.

## Discovery of HCV

*Hepatitis* simply means "inflammation of the liver." It is a combination of two words: "hepato" from the Greek *hepatikos,* meaning "liver," and "-itis," meaning "inflammation of." A great many things can cause inflammation in the liver: viruses, bacteria, chemicals, alcohol, and trauma. It's confusing, especially when the hepatitis alphabet diseases (hepatitis A through G) are discussed. The diseases sound related but they aren't. The structure, nature, and communicability of the viruses that cause each of them are very different. These viruses are all fairly new to human science: The hepatitis B virus (HBV) was isolated in 1965, HAV in 1973. HCV took a little longer to isolate.

Japanese researchers realized as early as the 1970s that an unknown pathogen was causing severe liver disease in their patients. The liver problems they were seeing could not be attributed to the A or B viruses. As it became clear that another distinct pathogen was involved, medical texts began referring to this new condition as "non-A, non-B" hepatitis. It was not until 1989 that the specific virus was isolated; shortly afterward it was genetically mapped by researchers in the United States. By 1991, a test for determining the presence of HCV antibodies had been created (from the blood of an Australian aborigine whose people have, disturbingly, never received reimbursement for their contribution), thereby allowing blood supplies around the world to be tested for the presence of the virus. Until that time, there was no way to determine whether blood supplies used for transfusions were contaminated. And many were.

## Spread by Infected Blood

The spread of the virus got a boost during and after World War II, as blood transfusions became common. Asian, African, American, and European blood supplies were liberally mixed during and immediately after the war as technological medicine was spread throughout those areas for the treatment of injured and displaced populations. This extensively spread the virus in human populations throughout the world (the 1940s — the First Wave). As soldiers and displaced people returned home, the widespread use of vaccines, needles, blood donation, and various surgical procedures (from dental visits to cesarean sections) helped spread the virus throughout the general population of each country (the 1950s and '60s — the Second Wave). Intravenous drug use, needle sharing, and contaminated blood banks (some addicts sell their blood weekly to get money for drugs) spread the virus even further (the 1970s and '80s — the Third Wave).

Because HCV is a relatively benign and slow-acting virus in its initial effects on the body (it rarely causes acute disease symptoms or discomfort at the time of infection), it takes a long time to notice. The disease really wasn't recognized until the late 1960s and early 1970s, when people contaminated in the First Wave began to show signs of liver disease. It is estimated that one-twelfth of the world population, or 500 million people, is now infected with HCV. In comparison, HIV infects 33 million people worldwide.

## THE HEPATITIS B VIRUS

The hepatitis B virus (HBV) was identified in 1965. HBV is transmitted from mother to child in utero and through sex, infected medical instruments, infected blood, and needle sharing. The onset of disease is often acute, as with hepatitis A, and can be severe. However, hepatitis B is not often fatal. Only about 7 percent of adults fail to clear the virus from the blood on their own and become chronic carriers. The outcome for chronic HBV infection is similar to that for chronic HCV infection.

HBV is a relatively stable DNA virus, a characteristic that has facilitated the development of a vaccine. The vaccine has many problems, and its use in young infants, although strongly recommended by physicians, carries potentially great health risks. Older children and adults can experience side effects ranging from mild to severe. All side effects should be considered before the vaccine is used. Co-infection with HBV does not seem to present any greater risk to patients who also have HCV infection. Some evidence suggests that HCV suppresses the activity of HBV, making the latter less active during infection.

# UNDERSTANDING VIRUSES

Viruses, unlike bacteria, have no nucleus and no cell wall. They are the barest of life-forms honed to structural simplicity. Although there are many kinds of viruses, a virus is generally a strand of DNA or RNA surrounded by a mathematically elegant polyhedron, called a capsid, whose shape is virus specific. The capsid in turn is often surrounded by one or more protein envelopes. The surface of the virus's protein envelope is studded with receptors. These receptors are actually sensory organs that tell the virus about its surroundings and are designed to help the virus find the particular kinds of cells it can live within.

## Classifications of Viruses

Viruses are typed in many ways: by size or shape, presence or absence of an enclosing capsule (not all viruses have one), whether they are DNA or RNA based (and from that, whether they are single or double stranded, positive or negative sense), their type of protein structure, and their manner of replication. DNA viruses are fairly reliable as viruses go because they have a kind of "copy-check" mechanism that RNA viruses lack. This means that when a DNA virus is making more of itself within a "borrowed" cell, it uses a biofeedback loop to make sure that the copies of itself are reasonably accurate. In contrast, an RNA virus is missing the gene structure that would allow it to do this. It tends to make a whole lot of copies that vary, sometimes a great deal, from the original. Growing evidence suggests that some of these copy differences are intentionally initiated by RNA viruses to increase their genetic variation and, hence, survivability.

Thus, while it is often possible to come up with a vaccine for a DNA virus, it can be

> "Viruses have a kind of sensation that could be classed as intermediate between a rudimentary smell or touch. . . . They have a way of detecting the chemical composition of cell surfaces. . . . This gives a virus the most exquisite ability to sense the right cell surfaces [allowing it to find its unique host cell]. It recognizes them through a perception in three-dimensional surface chemistry."
>
> — FRANK RYAN, MD, *Virus X: Tracking the New Killer Plagues*

difficult to make one for an RNA virus. This also makes RNA viruses very hard to treat with pharmaceutical agents; like bacteria, these viruses begin creating solutions to synthetic drugs the moment they encounter one. (Early evidence indicates that the mutation rate of HCV accelerates in response to interferon and ribavirin therapy, much as bacteria do with antibiotics.) Infection with an RNA virus such as HCV is actually quite different from infection with a DNA virus.

Whereas DNA viruses make billions of copies of themselves, RNA viruses make billions of similar but not identical viruses. It is something like a swarm of honeybees — all similar but all different. In fact, it is much more accurate to think of an RNA infection as infection by a viral swarm. The ones most similar to each other are the ones that die off when the human immune system is first activated or a pharmaceutical drug that can recognize them is used. This leaves the others free to multiply unchecked, and they multiply very fast indeed (some viruses produce a new generation every minute) while still making subtle changes in each new virus produced. HCV replicates extremely rapidly.

Evidence also indicates that both DNA and RNA viruses, like bacteria, share information between themselves in order to remain unaffected by medical treatments or immune systems. Similar viruses will actively share genetic structure to create difficult-to-treat infections. The common influenza virus, for instance, specifically and intentionally both rearranges its genetic structure and inserts entirely new genes within itself on a regular basis to remain invisible to the human immune system. (It gets these new gene sequences from birds in Asia.) This is why a new vaccine is needed every year for the flu.

### How They Infect

When not in a living cell, viruses go into a state of hibernation. In this state of dormancy, they move with air currents or in water, or they simply rest dormant on the ground until they come into contact with a life-form that contains the cells they need to awaken from their long sleep. At that moment, a virus's first tasks are to get inside the new host organism, to bypass its protective mechanisms, and to find the proper host cell. Many researchers now feel that viruses use what they call a genomic intelligence (as do bacteria) to solve the problems they face;

they actually begin experimenting with new combinations of genes to solve problems. In some instances, they actually have self-designed their genetic structure in such a way as to facilitate entry into new host organisms. (The rabies virus, for instance, causes uncontrolled biting at the same time that it swarms by the billions into the saliva of infected animals. Every time the animal bites something, the virus enters a new host.)

Once inside a new host organism, a virus, through the receptors on its protein envelope, begins seeking out cells in which it can live. Sometimes it simply circulates in the new organism's internal fluids until chance brings it into contact with the cells it is looking for. But in many instances, a virus uses the organism's own immune system to help because the cells it is looking for are a part of that same immune system. Such is the case with HIV, which views CD4 T lymphocytes as the perfect host cell; the Epstein-Barr virus, which has an affinity for human B cells; or even HCV, which loves liver cells (hepatocytes), lymphocytes, and monocytes.

As soon as the proper cell comes into contact with the virus, the virus sticks to it. The receptors on the surface of the virus fool the cell into thinking that the virus is a compatible protein that has attached, and the cell lets the virus inside. As soon as this happens, the virus sheds its protein coat and begins taking over the cell. (Sometimes, as with HIV, it will even insert itself into the host cell's DNA structure, from which it is very difficult to remove.) Eventually the cell is full of viruses, and it bulges outward and breaks open. As the viruses stream out of the dying cell, they take up parts of the cell membrane and make themselves new viral protein coats with receptors for new host cells.

Thus, the ancient struggle begins: finding out which is in better shape — the organism's immune system or the replicating virus. If the virus is particularly strong or if the immune system is compromised in any way, disease is often inevitable.

## AN INSIDE VIEW OF HCV

Magnified, HCV looks a lot like a mathematically elegant soccer ball. This "soccer ball" is the capsid, the protective covering of the virus. It is surrounded by two protein envelopes. Inside all this, kept safe from the perils of the outside world, is a single-stranded, positive-sense sequence of RNA, the HCV virus itself. Once inside a proper host cell, this strand of RNA immediately goes to the ribosomes or manufacturing centers of the cell and takes over.

### Producing a Viral Swarm

Because DNA is so large, it stays within the nucleus of our cells. It makes small RNA strands of genes, coded for particular manufacturing tasks, and sends them to the ribosomes. When the ribosomes encounter HCV RNA, they think it is a message from the cell's own DNA. The message the ribosome has received is "make lots and lots of copies of this genetic sequence." Unfortunately for the cell the genetic sequence is HCV RNA. As these copies are made, slight changes occur in the section of the RNA sequence that contains instructions for creating the protein coat and capsid that surround the virus. This means that when the new viruses leave the cell, they will all be slightly different than the parent virus. A viral swarm is now present in the body.

## THE HEPATITIS D, E, AND G VIRUSES

The hepatitis D virus (HDV) is found only in hepatitis B carriers, and it needs HBV to replicate. Co-infection with HBV and HDV can result in severe liver damage and chronic liver disease.

The hepatitis E virus (HVE), caused by a waterborne calcivirus, causes disease similar to hepatitis A and is transmitted similarly. It is usually found in developing countries.

Hepatitis G is also known as GBV. It was isolated from a surgeon (whose initials were GB) who was experiencing acute icteric hepatitis, and it was found to be distinct from all other hepatitis viruses. When injected into primates, it caused infection. One and a half percent of blood donors in London are infected with this form of hepatitis. Early projections show that up to 20 percent of patients with hepatitis C may be co-infected with it. There is no easy test for it, although a polymerase chain reaction (PCR) test can be performed (see appendix 1). It is unknown how severely this virus might affect human health or people infected with other hepatitis viruses.

### Establishing Itself in the Cells

At the same time the viral swarm is being created, the cell's ribosomes have also been instructed to make a special protein that goes immediately to the nucleus of the cell to make sure that the cell doesn't commit suicide. Normally, when cells are infected by viruses, they immediately begin to self-destruct, engaging in a process called apoptosis. During apoptosis, the cell releases a type of interferon that instructs all the nearby cells to also die (and also instructs the immune system to become more active) to remove usable host cells from the vicinity of the virus. Many viruses, HCV among them, have developed techniques to interfere with apoptosis. One of these involves the ability of the protein that keeps the cell alive. This allows HCV to spread through the body to the blood, lymph system, liver, and cerebrospinal fluid. At this point it becomes systemically entrenched, and a person has chronic HCV infection. Once this occurs, even if the virus is cleared from the blood, it will usually be present in other parts of the body. New research has also located HCV in bone marrow, kidney monocytes, B lymphocytes, and granulocytes.

## HCV'S FAMILY TREE

Because of its genetic structure, HCV is considered a member of the family Flaviviridae, which currently includes flaviviruses, carmoviruses, pestiviruses, and hepaciviruses (HCV belongs to this group). Hepatitis A, in comparison, is a picornavirus, not even close to HCV in its genetic structure.

The flaviviruses include tick-borne encephalitis, dengue virus serotype 4, yellow fever virus (which also infects the liver and causes a yellowing of the skin and eyes called jaundice), and the West Nile virus, which recently infected New York City (see Epilogue). The carmoviruses infect specific plants: carnations, turnips, maize, barley, red clover, cucumbers, and tomatoes. The pestiviruses include bovine viral diarrhea virus and swine fever virus.

Because HCV is similar to both animal-infective and plant-infective viruses (it contains genetic sequences from both), many researchers feel that HCV is an evolutionary link between plant and animal viruses. As such, it would be one of the first viruses identified that shares genetic material between plants and animals (see Epilogue). Because HCV was so recently identified — only a decade ago — its original host has not yet been identified. HCV has been found only in humans and intentionally infected chimpanzees.

## Major Strains

As with many viruses, it turns out that HCV's primary genetic structure is slightly altered depending on the geographical area in which it is found. Six major types or strains and some 60 subtypes have been located. Of these, the most aggressive seems to be type 1, subtype b (type 1b). This type responds the most poorly of all strains to interferon and ribavirin. It is the most common type in the United States, Japan, and Europe.

In general, type 1 (and its corresponding subtypes) is predominant in the Americas, Europe, India, Australia, and Russia; it is common nearly everywhere. Type 2 is predominant in Italy and common in China, Japan, Taiwan, and Indonesia; and type 3 is predominant in Thailand and common in the United Kingdom, Australia, Sweden, India, and Brazil. Type 4 is predominant in western Africa and is common in the Middle East. Type 5 is predominant in South Africa, and type 6 is predominant in Hong Kong and Macao and common in Vietnam. Although it is possible to test a person for a particular type of HCV, testing is very rarely done because of the cost.

## Tracing Its Path

As researchers began to understand the virus and watch its growth patterns, they could tell how much genetic drift occurs during replication; that is, how much the virus differs from its parent as it replicates. They then used mathematical projection to estimate how long it has taken for the major strains of HCV to form from an original parent virus and from which part of Earth it first entered humans.

From genetic drift, it appears that HCV encountered the human species about 200 years ago in the Far East. From that original encounter it was carried to West Africa, India, and southeast Asia, where the greatest diversity of HCV subtypes now exists. Although this information may be refined further as new data are encountered, the current picture does make sense. The 1790s were a period of exhaustive exploration. Significant long-distance travel was occurring between the continents, and after the initial insertion of HCV into humans the virus could then be easily carried on trade routes, much as bubonic plague (caused by the *Yersinia pestis* bacterium, which is carried in fleas and spread by flea-infested rodents) and other diseases had traveled in the past. And like infection with *Y. pestis,* the spread of HCV has reached plague proportions in the 200 years in which the virus has intermixed with the human species. It is one of the most widely spread serious diseases on Earth.

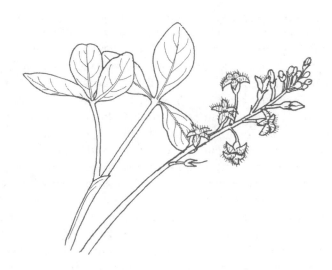

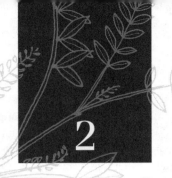

# HEPATITIS C, THE LIVER, AND THE IMMUNE SYSTEM

As hepatitis C progresses, it begins to disrupt the elegant and balanced ecosystem of the human body. Because liver and immune cells are its primary host cells, these are the cells that tend to suffer most from the presence of the virus. Eventually, as more and more liver cells are disrupted, the liver itself can begin to fail. This leads to many of the problems associated with hepatitis C liver disease.

The liver performs an amazing array of complex functions to keep us healthy. It converts food into energy, deactivates any toxic substances we breathe and eat, absorbs and processes fats and vitamins, and creates many hormones, enzymes, amino acids, and proteins that are essential for health. One of its major jobs is to clear the blood of toxins; it is in essence a kind of filter through which 2¼ pints (1.2 L) of blood flow per minute. The better the liver works, the more toxins are processed and the better we feel. This filtering process makes it one of the major components of our immune system. (This is also how HCV finds its liver host cells, traveling in the blood as a part of the body's normal cleansing process.)

## THE LIVER AND THE IMMUNE SYSTEM

The progenitor of all immune cells, the stem cell, is made in our bone marrow. Many stem cells turn into monocytes, which, in turn, can become macrophages, whose main job is to continually search the body and "eat" anything they find that is toxic or foreign. The liver contains a large, permanent concentration of macrophages (they make up about 10 percent of liver tissue) called the Kupffer cells. These cells "eat" or process the toxins and foreign particles that are brought to the liver through the blood. This includes viruses. But viruses are actually too small to be "seen" by Kupffer cells and, in general, can't be "eaten" without first being processed by other parts of the immune system.

### Immune Cells

Stem cells can become a wide variety of immune cells: eosinophils, neutrophils, basophils, mast cells, monocytes, macrophages, plasma cells, B cells, and 11 different kinds of T cells. Each immune cell has its own specialized function.

T cell actually means "thymus cell" because stem cells are processed in the thymus gland to become T cells. As a result, it's crucial to support thymus health in chronic viral diseases such as HCV infection. (Researchers have also shown that people with higher numbers of one kind of T cell [so-called T-helper cells, or CD4+] have much less severe liver damage from HCV.) B cells primarily work to produce antibodies; T cells perform many functions, including the release of interleukin-2 (which stimulates T-cell production and tells B cells to begin producing antibodies) and interferon-alpha (which speeds up and regulates the response of immune cells to the invader).

### Antibodies

Although macrophages can and do just happen upon protein-coated viruses and eat them, these viruses are hard for macrophages to detect. Thus, the immune system produces antibodies; a lot of them are produced by the B cells. Antibodies are tiny recognition structures (almost like viruses themselves) whose purpose is to encircle specific chemical structures. They actually make a cage that imprisons the virus. This cage and its contents (called an antigen–antibody complex) is big enough to be seen and processed by the body's immune system. As the blood circulates through the liver, the Kupffer cells consume and process the constituents of antigen–antibody complexes.

## WHAT IS THE LIVER?

In many respects, the liver is simply transformed blood (it contains only 4 percent less fluid than blood itself); it is the largest reservoir of blood in the body and is the body's warmest organ. It looks much like calf's liver, is tucked under the right rib cage, and, in adults, weighs 2½ to 3 pounds (1–1¼ kg). Unless the liver is inflamed, only a centimeter or so projects down from under the rib cage.

The liver consists of two primary lobes (the right and left lobe), each of which can function independently. In turn, each lobe contains up to 50,000 tiny lobules. These are the functional units of the liver; they do all the work. Each has a vein, artery, lymph channel, and bile channel.

---

### LIVER REGENERATION

The liver is the only organ of the body that can regenerate. Up to 75 percent of the liver can be removed, and within 2 or 3 months the liver will regrow to its original shape and size. This has been known for thousands of years in western traditions of healing. In one ancient Greek legend, Prometheus was punished for bringing fire to humankind. He was chained to a rock, and each day vultures fed on his liver, which then regenerated each night.

---

### The Filtering Process

The liver receives oxygenated blood from the heart through the hepatic artery but receives "used" blood through the portal vein. The portal vein carries all the blood from the stomach, pancreas, spleen, and intestines (filled with substances removed from our food), and this blood is filtered through the liver before returning to the heart and lungs for reoxygenation. The usable bits are processed as fuel, building blocks, and essential nutrients, and the toxins are broken down to essential components and used or packaged for removal. (Many synthetic chemicals — we are exposed to thousands of them each day — are so unusual that the liver cannot figure out what to do with them and thus simply stores them, often in fat tissue.) The gallbladder and bile ducts collect bile from the thousands of lobules of the liver. Excess bile is stored in the gallbladder and is released after meals so that it can help in digestion.

## ALL ABOUT BILE

Bile is composed of bile salts, cholesterol, and bile pigments (with a pinch of lecithin, mucin, and alkali carbonates); it is very bitter. To make it, the liver culls old red blood cells and breaks them down into two "pigments" or components: bilirubin and biliverdin. These are combined with another chemical to make them soluble in water. The colors of the bile pigments are yellow and green.

### Bile Pigments

Bile pigments give feces their distinctive color. If the bile ducts are blocked, bile cannot get to the intestines and the feces become pale and, in extreme cases, white. In the bowel, bilirubin is converted to urobilinogen, which is reabsorbed and excreted through the kidneys, giving urine its characteristic yellow color. If the bilirubin cannot get out through the gallbladder (or if too much is produced or the liver is damaged, as in hepatitis), it passes into the bloodstream, raising bilirubin levels in the blood. This can lead to jaundice (a yellowing of the skin and eyes) and to "tea-colored" urine. Sometimes bile salts are also deposited in the skin, which causes itching (pruritus); this is a very common symptom in hepatitis C and liver disease.

### What Color Is Your Bruise?

You can see bile pigment colors in a bruise. As the damaged blood spreads out in the skin tissue, it is broken down by liver enzymes into bilirubin and biliverdin. Thus, as the bruise "heals," it changes from the red/blue of blood cells to green and yellow as the liver enzymes break down the blood cells. Finally, the bruise disappears as the blood cells are reabsorbed into the system.

### Bile Salts

Bile salts are made by the liver from cholesterol and are used over and over again. They are responsible for emulsifying fats and fat-soluble vitamins in the intestines and bringing them back to the liver for processing. They also dissolve cholesterol to keep it in solution for use by the body. If insufficient bile salts are being produced, then cholesterol will begin to precipitate out in the gallbladder as gallstones. In liver disease and HCV infection, bile production is insufficient and bile movement is sluggish. In this condition, called cholestasis, essential nutrients to maintain bodily health are not taken up in solution in the quantities needed and those that are taken up are not transported quickly enough.

## UNDERSTANDING THE LIVER'S CYCLE AND CHALLENGES WITH HCV

All organs in the body, and the body itself, tend to have certain periodic cycles to their functioning. Brain waves are very fast, the menstrual cycle is very slow. The liver cycles every 24 hours.

The liver synthesizes complex chemicals and processes toxins the most when the production of bile is lowest, and vice versa. Because bile is needed for food processing, our bodies make a lot of it during the day and not very much at night. (This is why a big meal at night isn't good for the body; the liver isn't designed to deal with it.) Bile production is highest at 9 A.M. and lowest at 9 P.M. During the late evening and night, the liver converts to its other function, that of synthesizing complex chemicals and processing the day's accumulated toxins. This process peaks around 9 P.M. and is lowest at 9 A.M.

People with liver disease are often so sensitive that, when this cycle begins shifting at 3 A.M., they wake up from their sleep. (At this time, the liver starts slowing synthesis and readying itself for bile production; this happens again at 3 P.M.; at that point, synthesis starts to increase and bile decreases). When people with liver disease wake up at 3 A.M., they are often deeply depressed and, despite the general fatigue that HCV infection causes, can't go back to sleep. The mind begins to race, turning melancholic thoughts over and over. (Melancholy was recognized by the ancients as a symptom of liver disease. It means "black bile" and comes in part from the liver's inability to synthesize many of the necessary hormones needed for well-being.)

It is very important that patients with HCV infection (and all liver diseases) orient

> "Liver-based fatigue produces a terrible sense of lifelessness and a loss of will. With the sapping of the will comes impairment of the ability for forethought. Exhaustion can become too overmastering that getting out of bed to begin the day requires monumental effort."
>
> —JESSE STOFF, MD COAUTHOR, *Chronic Fatigue Syndrome: The Hidden Epidemic*

sleeping (by going to bed at 9 P.M.) and treatment (by taking herbs and supplements just before bed) around this natural rhythm of the liver to facilitate sleep, decrease depression, and help the liver process accumulated toxins and synthesize and process needed chemicals. Many of these necessary chemicals are processed from the food we eat, usually through the conversion of protein, carbohydrates, and fats.

## Protein Breakdown

Meat, fish, nuts, dairy products (such as cheese, milk, and eggs), and certain plants, such as beans and seaweeds, are the major sources of protein in the human diet. The liver, through the action of bile in the intestines, breaks proteins down into the 22 amino acids needed to maintain the cells and tissues in our bodies. Ten of these amino acids are "essential," meaning that they must come from outside our bodies in our food. The remaining amino acids are synthesized, primarily by the liver, from the original ten. These amino acids are the building blocks of our body and are used to repair damaged DNA and cellular tissue.

The liver damage caused by HCV makes it difficult for the liver to engage in protein synthesis and to synthesize the amino acids we need. This results in protein and amino acid deficiencies. In just one example, albumin is generated from proteins by the liver and is usually present in high quantities in the blood. Albumin helps regulate the fluid balance in cells; prevents cell mutation (thus helping prevent cancer); scavenges stress hormones; removes waste products from connective tissue; transports vitamins, minerals, and fatty acids throughout the body; aids general liver function; and helps deactivate chemical toxins. Low albumin levels in the blood are a sign of liver disease. HCV infection and liver disease prevent or slow this process of protein conversion and essentially produce a form of malnutrition.

## Carbohydrate Conversion

Sugar and starch are the main sources of carbohydrates in our diets and are converted into glucose, which is more easily usable by the body. The liver converts excess glucose into glycogen, which is stored in the liver and muscles; it is reconverted back to glucose whenever more energy is needed. One of the symptoms of HCV infection and liver disease is either too much or not enough sugar in the blood (this results in hyperglycemia or hypoglycemia.) Another is fatigue caused in part by the liver's inability to process glucose and glycogen effectively. When you need fuel (glucose), the liver can't utilize it fast enough and you literally run out of gas.

### Fat Breakdown

Fat is one of the best sources of energy available. One gram of fat provides 9 calories of energy; carbohydrates or proteins provide only 4. Fats are broken down in the liver for use as calories of energy and for use as specific kinds of fats, such as cholesterol and triglycerides. The liver and body need these to carry out many of their functions.

During HCV infection, LDL (low-density lipoprotein) — the "bad" cholesterol — tends to build up in the system, and HDL (high-density lipoprotein) — the "good" cholesterol — tends to decrease. Overall, serum cholesterol levels in the blood tend to increase, leading to increased risk of heart disease and stroke. Levels of other fats in the blood, such as triglycerides, also increase.

Hepatitis C and other liver diseases can also cause fatty deposits in the liver, a condition called fatty liver or steatosis, which can result in cirrhosis and produces many of the symptoms of hepatitis. If the liver is having trouble processing fats, people often start feeling an aversion to eating fat of any kind. Consumption of fat in such circumstances can result in a feeling of "biliousness," a unique kind of nausea. The word means "a condition caused by an excess of bile."

### Hormones and Enzymes

The liver continually synthesizes many important hormones and enzymes, all of which are affected by liver disease. Others, synthesized elsewhere in the body, are used extensively by the liver to carry out its detoxifying and synthesizing functions. One of the most important is glutathione, synthesized in the mitochondria and normally present in large amounts in the liver. Glutathione production is dependent on the amino acids cysteine and glutamic acid, which the liver must process from our food. Glutathione is perhaps the most powerful substance for detoxification and maintenance of cell health. More important, recent research has shown that glutathione is an exceptionally powerful antiviral.

When present in normal amounts it strongly inhibits viral replication. Reduced levels of glutathione allow unrestrained growth of whatever viruses are present in the body. Recent studies have shown that HIV, HCV, Epstein-Barr, and possibly HHV6 all contain gene sequences that specifically reduce glutathione levels in the body. Studies have also shown that low glutathione leads to premature aging, numerous chronic and degenerative diseases, and the inability of the liver to process toxins.

The liver also helps process many sexual hormones. Some of the symptoms of improper processing are loss of libido, menstrual irregularity, impotence, loss of body hair, and severe mood swings.

## CIRRHOSIS AND HCV

During advanced HCV infection, cirrhosis can develop from two processes. The first is directly caused by HCV itself. As the virus takes over, more and more cells in the liver die either from apoptosis or from the virus exploding out of the cell as it makes more of itself. The second is caused by the human immune system. As lymphocytes rush to the liver to attack the virus, the body's liver cells are often damaged or destroyed in the process. The bile duct is often damaged and scarred, which can be the source of liver pain. As the disease progresses, instead of the liver regenerating as smooth liver tissue, the liver forms lumpy nodules and scar tissue instead — cirrhosis. This means that as the damage spreads, fewer and fewer healthy liver cells are available to process blood. The same amount of blood is trying to be filtered through the liver, but there are not enough cells available to process it.

At this point, the liver increasingly fails to do its many tasks, and blood from the portal vein begins to back up. This blood creates pressure by trying to get in where there is nowhere for it to go. Many symptoms are associated with this: portal hypertension (elevated blood pressure caused by portal congestion), fluid retention in the lower extremities, and ascites.

### Related Diseases

Other diseases that can occur as a manifestation of HCV infection are membranoproliferative glomerulonephritis, essential mixed cryo-globulinemia, porphyria cutanea tarda, leukocyto-clastic vasculitis, focal lymphocytic sialadenitis, Mooren corneal ulcers, lichen planus, idiopathic pulmonary fibrosis, and rheumatoid arthritis.

Ascites is fluid in the abdominal cavity. It is caused by the pressure in the portal vein. The red blood cells are too large to be pushed through the walls of the veins, but the blood plasma is not. It is pushed out into the space surrounding the intestines, the peritoneal cavity. This cavity can eventually hold up to 10 quarts (10 L) of liquid. A rather large "beer belly" forms. It is usually painless, although the patient often feels a sense of fullness, and it can hurt if the amount of liquid begins to press on other internal organs. Physicians sometimes stick a needle in the abdominal cavity and draw off the fluid or prescribe diuretics.

## HEALING OF LIVER DISEASE AND HEPATITIS C

Fortunately, many of the traditional herbal medicines used for liver disease throughout the world have been found to be exceptionally effective for treatment of hepatitis C. Herbal clinicians and scientific researchers exploring herbal approaches to HCV infection in vitro, in vivo, and in human trials all note that herbal medicines show exceptional strength in reversing the course of the disease. They have also reported that in a majority of patients, symptoms resolve, liver enzyme levels normalize, and viral load often disappears. As Matthew Dolan comments in *The Hepatitis C Handbook:*

> Austrian research suggests that a similar result [to certain expensive and side-effect laden experimental pharmaceuticals] can be achieved using antiviral herbs; however there is an interesting difference in the profile of the decline in the viral load. Herbal treatment appears to achieve a slower but steadier decline in the viral load, indicating that it is penetrating into the "compartments," and neutralizing the virus in longer lived cells; in other words, it reaches the parts that antiviral drugs cannot reach.

The following chapters outline a five-part protocol and explore the herbs and foods that have been found to be exceptionally effective for treatment of hepatitis C. Chapter 7 outlines several versions of the protocol itself so that it can be easily followed on a daily basis; it also contains a listing of herbs found useful for some of the specific symptoms associated with HCV infection.

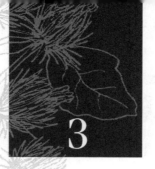

# BOTANICAL MEDICINES
# FOR HEPATITIS C
# AND THE LIVER

At a recent conference on naturopathic medicine, one of the speakers, a clinician, laughed and said (in response to someone earnestly talking about the importance of dandelion), "Well, nobody ever got hepatitis or liver disease from not eating dandelion." I laughed, too, at the time. Then I began to wonder.

Until World War II, the human diet was very different than it is now. In fact, dandelion was a regular part of the American diet and the diet of other peoples around the world. Throughout most of human history, people ate a great variety of plants — we grazed in a sense, much like herbivores still do. This extremely diverse diet included many potent medicinal plants. In fact, a great deal of evidence suggests that all animals, including humans, are drawn to different plants at different times to meet nutritional and medicinal needs. Not so oddly, then, many of the plants that are good for hepatitis are actually food plants once extremely common in human diets.

The intake of a rich variety of plants in our diets throughout our lives has strong effects on our liver functioning and overall health. In some respects, the increase of several diseases, including hepatitis, might correlate in part to the narrowing of our diets and the monocropping of our agricultural foods. In the past, humans might still have been infected with hepatitis viruses, but the normal diet would have contained scores of plants that potentiated liver functioning and resistance to liver disease, thus minimizing the effects of the disease.

# HERBS FOR THE LIVER

Scores of herbs have beneficial effects on the liver, have been used throughout time for healing liver disease (as foods and medicines), and have been found to be specifically active against hepatitis viruses. What follows is a subjective gathering of 10 of the strongest herbs. I have used three overlapping criteria to arrive at this list: length of and reputed efficacy in historical use, current recognition among clinicians of effectiveness in treating hepatitis C, and scientific studies — in vitro, in vivo, or human trials. In other words, these herbs

> ## A Note on References
>
> For ease of flow in the text, the literature citations are included in the Selected Bibliography. Information on how to make the various herbal preparations described is included in appendix 2.

have been successfully used for a long time by humans in the treatment of liver disease and inflammation, they are currently recognized by modern practitioners as being effective in the treatment of hepatitis and liver disease, and scientific studies have verified both historical and contemporary uses.

Many of these herbs stimulate production and flow of bile, which are essential in counteracting cholestasis; others protect the liver from harm; others help it regenerate; and still others act directly as antiviral agents against hepatitis viruses. Those that stimulate bile flow should not be used if there are obstructed bile ducts.

> ## Top 10 Botanical Medicines for Hepatitis C
>
> Baical skullcap
> Boldo
> Bupleurum
> Burdock
> Dandelion
> Milk thistle
> Phyllanthus
> Picrorhiza
> Reishi mushroom
> Turmeric

## Types of Actions

In general, three types of liver herbs should be used for treating hepatitis C: 1) herbs that reverse or prevent damage to liver cells, 2) herbs that possess antiviral action against hepatitis viruses, and 3) herbs that reverse hepatitis symptoms (such as high blood enzyme levels) and optimize liver functioning.

# BAICAL SKULLCAP *(Scutellaria baicalensis)*

**Family:** Labiatae.

**Part used:** Root.

**Collection and habitat:** Northern China, the mountains of southwestern China, Manchuria, and Siberia. Rare in Europe and the United States. Plants are harvested when they are 3 to 4 years old, usually in the spring. The roots are cleaned, dried under light sunshine until partly dry, then sliced and dried out of the sun until completely dry.

**Actions:** Hepatoprotective, antihepatotoxic, choleretic, anti-inflammatory, antioxidant, antipyretic, refrigerant, blood pressure–lowering (hypotensive), central nervous system sedative, antibacterial, antiviral, diuretic, bladder tonic, anodyne.

**Functions in liver disease:** Protects the liver from hepatic toxins, reduces inflammation in the liver, stimulates bile production, alleviates jaundice, alleviates sleep disorders associated with liver disease, and alleviates recurrent fevers and chills associated with hepatitis.

**Specific indications:** Intermittent fever, mental and physical exhaustion, wakefulness and restlessness, arthritis generated by liver disease.

## Uses of Baical Skullcap

This is a cousin of the common western herb known as skullcap. In traditional Chinese medicine, it has a reputation as a potent liver tonic and protector in addition to possessing the same central nervous system–relaxant qualities as western skullcap. The herb is fairly easy to find because it is regularly used in Chinese medicine in the United States.

**Ayurvedic:** Apparently unknown.

**Chinese:** Used in traditional Chinese medicine (TCM) for over 2000 years, baical skullcap is one of the regular ingredients in minor bupleurum combination (see bupleurum), a major TCM treatment formula for hepatitis. It is considered a bitter, cold herb with an affinity for the gallbladder, heart, lungs, and large and small intestines. It is called "huang qin" in TCM.

**Western botanic practice:** Western botanic practice has focused on other *Scutellaria* species, primarily *Scutellaria laterifolia*. Still, there is some overlap with baical skullcap in range of use. The eclectic botanic physicians of the 19th century found skullcap to be effective in helping alleviate intermittent fever, mental or physical exhaustion, wakeful-ness, and restlessness, especially if those conditions followed acute disease or accompanied chronic disease. This makes skullcap perfect for treating chronic hepatitis, in which such symptoms are common. Hepatoprotective activity is not generally recognized in western species of skullcap. The Chinese herb is entering western practice through the influence of TCM.

**Scientific:** Most of the clinical trials for hepatitis have focused on minor bupleurum combination, which contains baical skullcap. However, Steven Foster and Yue Chongxi note in their book *Herbal Emissaries* that "clinical studies [with baical skullcap] have indicated utility in chronic hepatitis, with over 70 percent effectiveness rate. Symptoms were improved, including an increase in appetite, relief of abdominal distention, and improved liver function." Foster goes on to note that one of the constituents in baical skullcap, baicalin, is used clinically in China (in intramuscularly injectable form) for treating acute and infectious hepatitis. Research studies and clinical reports support these actions of baical skullcap in liver disease and hepatitis. Baical skullcap has been found both in vivo and in vitro to be an effective antihepatotoxic herb. Studies show protection against liver damage induced by carbon tetrachloride ($CCl_4$), galactosamine, and acetaminophen. After dosing with the herb, liver enzyme levels tended to normalize and liver degeneration was halted. In one trial, when baical skullcap was combined with *Artemisia capillaris* and *Gardenia jasminoides,* fulminant hepatitis was successfully treated in vivo. Other studies have shown that the herb significantly increases bile production.

## Preparation and Dosage

May be used as tea or in capsules.

**Tea:** 3–9 grams powdered root in ½ ounce (15 mL) water. Bring to a boil, remove from heat, let steep 15–20 minutes. Drink 3 times per day.

**Capsules:** 2–4 "00" capsules of the powdered root 3 times a day.

## Contraindications and Side Effects

Contraindicated in obstructed bile duct. No side effects noted.

# BOLDO *(Peumus boldus)*

**Family:** Monimiaceae.
**Part used:** Leaf.
**Collection and habitat:** A South and Central American herb; it can be harvested at any time.
**Actions:** Hepatoanalgesic, hepatoprotective, antihepatotoxic, anti-inflammatory, choleretic, antioxidant, liver tonic, kidney tonic, antispasmodic, bitter, antibacterial, antifungal.
**Functions in liver disease:** Reducing liver pain and inflammation, protecting the liver from toxin damage, stimulating production of bile, alleviating jaundice, easing sleep disturbance, promoting and supporting healthy functioning of the kidneys (thus taking some of the load off the liver).
**Specific indications:** Liver pain, fatigue, sleep disorders.

## Uses of Boldo

Boldo grows extensively in Peru and Chile, although most of the commercial stocks come from Mexico. It is relatively inexpensive but sometimes can be hard to find. Several practitioners who have worked extensively with liver disease and hepatitis feel that boldo is the number one herb to use for active liver pain. Despite a dearth of current research, the clinicians who use the herb insist it is one of their most reliable herbs in the treatment of chronic liver disease.

**Ayurvedic:** Unknown.

**Chinese:** Unknown.

**Western botanic practice:** Boldo was limited to indigenous practice until 1875, when it was introduced into western practice by the eclectic botanic physicians. It was used irregularly until the fading of eclectic practice around 1935 and was forgotten until the past decade or so. Traditional South American use is for hepatic disease. Nineteenth-century western botanic practice focused on its uses as a liver tonic, for calming worry, and for easing sleep disturbances, gastric pain, and jaundice. It is officially approved in German medical practice and is listed in the German Commission E monographs for use in mild spastic problems of the gastrointestinal tract and dyspepsia.

**Scientific:** Boldo has undergone a limited number of scientific studies, primarily in Germany, France, and Chile. These initial studies have been highly promising. In vivo and in vitro studies have shown choleretic, antihepatotoxic, anti-inflammatory, antifungal, and antibacterial actions. One in vivo study in Chile of tert-butyl hydroperoxide–induced hepatotoxicity showed that lactate dehydrogenase and malondialdehyde levels and leakage of aminotransferase decreased. Boldo also protected against $CCl_4$-induced hepatotoxicity.

### Preparation and Dosage

May be used as tea or tincture or in capsules.
   **Tea:** 1 tsp (5 mL) in 6–8 ounces (180–240 mL) water, 3–4 times per day.
   **Tincture:** 1:5 60 percent alcohol; 5–20 drops up to 3 times per day.
   **Capsules:** 1–10 "00" capsules (up to 3 grams) per day.

### Contraindications and Side Effects

Contraindicated in obstructed bile duct.

## BUPLEURUM *(Bupleurum chinense* or *B. falcatum,* occasionally *B. fruticosum, B. kaoi)*

**Family:** Apiaceae.
**Part used:** In traditional medicine, the root; in two studies, however, the entire *B. chinense* plant was used and was found to be active in protecting against chemically induced hepatitis, $CCl_4$-induced hepatotoxicity, and acetaminophen-induced liver damage.
**Collection and habitat:** The plant grows primarily in China. The root should be dug in the fall and dried thoroughly in the shade.
**Actions:** Antipyretic, antihepatotoxic, antiviral, anticirrhotic, anti-inflammatory, hepatoprotective, hepatonormalizing, alterative, analgesic, immunostimulating, carminative, diaphoretic.
**Functions in liver disease:** Used to normalize liver function, retard liver damage, stimulate immune response (specifically, of antibody formation to hepatitis viruses and production and aggressiveness of white blood cells). It is viricidal against HBV and, it is thought, HCV. It is an excellent tonic when taken long term for viral hepatitis.

**Specific indications:** Viral hepatitis, elevated liver enzyme levels, intermittent fever and chills, advanced liver disease with resultant fatigue and malaise.

## Uses of Bupleurum

Bupleurum is a Chinese herb that, as far as I know, does not grow wild in the United States. It is fairly easy to find through herbal suppliers and health food stores.

**Ayurvedic:** Apparently unknown.

**Chinese:** Called "chai hu" in TCM; its common names are hare's ear, bupleuri root, and Chinese thoroughwax. Bupleurum is considered to be a neutral bitter with an affinity for the pericardium, liver, and gallbladder. It is one of the major components in minor bupleurum combination (also known as shosaikoto). This traditional Chinese formulation has been extensively tested in China and Japan in the treatment of viral hepatitis, and the results have been excellent (see Scientific uses). The herbs used in minor bupleurum combination can vary from practitioner to practitioner, but the following mixture is the one used in human clinical trials.

Minor bupleurum combination is composed of 7 parts bupleurum; 5 parts half summer root *(Pinellia ternata)*; 3 parts each ginseng *(Panax ginseng)*, Chinese skullcap root *(Scutellaria baicalensis),* and jujube fruit *(Zizyphus jujuba)*; 2 parts licorice root *(Glycyrrhiza glabra)*; and 1 part ginger root *(Zingeber officinalis)* — 24 parts total. In the scientific studies, the combination was given as a hot tea/infusion made from 7 g bupleurum, 2 g licorice root, 3 g jujube fruit, 1 g ginger root, 3 g ginseng, 3 g Chinese skullcap root, and 5 g half summer root (24 g total, about ¾ ounce) in 22 ounces (700 mL) water consumed throughout the day. Tea was taken for 1 month.

Minor bupleurum combination has traditionally been used for malaria and all conditions in which the presenting symptoms are intermittent fever and chills, fatigue, and weakness in the liver.

**Western botanic practice:** Unknown until recently. Introduced through TCM. Considered by a majority of western clinicians to be one of the best herbs for hepatitis.

**Scientific:** Bupleurum has been tested in at least 37 studies and has been found to have strong liver protective, antihepatotoxic, and antiviral activity for hepatitis viruses (in vivo, in vitro, or in human trials). The studies have generally taken place in Indonesia, Taiwan, China, South Korea, Japan, and Spain. Although the two species most commonly used are *B. chinense* and *B. falcatum,* other species have traditionally been used for the same kinds of liver symptoms and have been found in clinical trial to also be liver protective. *B. falcatum* has been reported to be directly antiviral against HBV.

Bupleurum has been found to be liver protective against hepatotoxicity induced by $CCl_4$, acetaminophen, and beta-D-galactosamine. *B. chinense* was found to protect the liver from fatty liver degeneration (steatosis) and to prevent necrosis. In one in vivo study, *B. falcatum* normalized liver function in $CCl_4$-induced liver damage in rats, as indicated by serum alkaline phosphatase levels and the retention of bromsulphalein. A combination of bupleurum and ginseng saponins given to mice before injection of $CCl_4$ was found to reduce cellular-level liver damage.

Minor bupleurum combination has undergone several studies, especially in Japan. One study of 13 patients with chronic hepatitis older than age 62 found that serum aspartate and alanine aminotransferase levels dropped. Another study found that the combination suppressed hyaline degeneration of the liver (galactosamine induced) and suppressed decrease in hepatic glutamine synthetase activity. The amount of minor bupleurum combination used for these studies was 5 g per day, given as a tea.

Minor bupleurum combination has been found to be antihepatotoxic and effective in the treatment of viral hepatitis. In one clinical trial, it promoted clearance of the hepatitis B surface antigen (HBsAg) in children with chronic HBV infection and sustained liver disease. Seven of 14 patients became HBsAg negative within 3 to 10 months. An experimental double-blind study of 222 patients with chronic hepatitis (116 received minor bupleurum combination and 106 received a placebo) found that serum aspartate aminotransferase and alanine aminotransferase values decreased significantly with 12-week administration of minor bupleurum combination. In patients with diagnosed HBV infection, HBsAg decreased and antihepatitis B antibodies increased. These responses apparently extend to HCV and HAV.

Minor bupleurum combination has shown significant immunostimulant activity and anti-inflammatory activity, the ability to prevent liver fibrosis, and the ability to increase interleukin production in peripheral blood mononuclear cells. Saikosaponin, one of the major constituents of bupleurum root, has been shown to increase antibody response, macrophage spreading, and phagocytosis in vivo.

Most studies used hot-water extracts (strong tea). Dosages varied. All the herbs in minor bupleurum combination have been found to have liver protective and anti-inflammatory actions in separate studies.

## Preparation and Dosage

As powder, capsules, or tea.

**Powder:** 1–2 tsp (2–5 g) per day.

**Capsules:** 4–10 "00" capsules daily (see Contraindications).

**Tea:** 1 tsp (5 mL) herb in 8 ounces (240 mL) hot water; strain and drink 3 times per day.

## Contraindications and Side Effects

May cause headache, anger, or nausea in some people. In such cases, the dose should be lowered (begin with low dose and work up). Otherwise, no side effects or contraindications have been noted.

## BURDOCK *(Arctium lappa)*

**Family:** Compositae.

**Part used:** The root and seed are used; the leaves are also used in Asia and were once commonly used in western practice.

**Collection and habitat:** Originally European, burdock is a biennial plant now naturalized throughout the world. The root should be picked at the end of the first year (preferably) or in early spring of the second year, just as the leaves are coming up; the seeds are ready for picking in late summer or early fall. The root is more commonly used in liver disease than the seeds.

**Actions:** Alterative, diuretic, bitter, anti-inflammatory, cholagogue, aperient, sudorific, antitumor.

**Functions in liver disease:** A broad-spectrum alterative to move the whole body and internal organs to a balanced state of health, especially for balancing and restoring the liver, lymph system, and kidneys. Useful in hepatic skin conditions: itching, eczema, dandruff, psoriasis, dry and scaly skin, skin eruptions, and increased cholesterol and LDL levels (see Scientific uses). The diuretic action of the seeds helps promote waste elimination as the kidneys take some of the burden off the liver.

**Specific indications:** Root — long-term chronic liver disease, poor skin condition, skin eruptions, high cholesterol levels, liver cancer. Seeds — fluid buildup related to liver disease, ascites, kidney weakness.

## Uses of Burdock

Burdock is known throughout the world as both a food and a medicinal herb. The grape-sized seed pods have the annoying habit of attaching themselves to anything and everything and being uncooperative about letting go. They were, in fact, the inspiration for the invention of Velcro.

The root is thought by many to be better if used fresh. Almost all Asian markets (and some health food stores) carry it as a normal food staple; thus, it is fairly easy to find fresh and can be prepared as food or medicinal herb. The stems can also be eaten and are delicious in stews and soups. The steamed root tastes much like a mild asparagus.

**Ayurvedic:** Apparently unknown.

**Chinese:** Called "niu bang zi" in China. The seeds and sometimes the root have a long history of use as an antitoxic herb (for cleansing the body of built-up toxins, as a blood cleanser), and as an antipyretic, antiphlogistic, and diuretic. The herb is considered a cold herb in Chinese medicine and thus is good for a hot, inflamed condition, such as hepatitis. Some of the specific indications for its use in TCM are throat infections, pneumonia, urinary tract infection, and abscesses. The seed tincture is considered especially potent in the topical treatment of psoriasis, hemorrhoids, and chronic sores.

**Western botanic practice:** Burdock has been used extensively in the West since at least the time of Dioscorides. Perhaps the best overall discussion of its uses and place in western herbalism is Matthew Wood's excellent *The Book of Herbal Wisdom,* wherein the author traces its use over two millennia. In short, he notes that "[burdock] seems to act particularly through the liver, lymphatics, and kidneys. It stimulates metabolism through the liver, cleansing and feeding through the lymph, and waste removal through the veins."

Traditionally, burdock was recognized more for its effects as a diuretic and helping the kidneys process waste and "re-tone" and for its actions in helping clear up difficult skin conditions, from boils to acne to psoriasis to eczema — in general, any active inflammation or eruption of the skin due to some underlying chronic condition. The recognition of its strong actions on the liver and lymphatic system came later, but these actions are firmly established today in western practice. Usually the herb is used with chronic conditions that affect the liver, kidneys, and lymph system. The seeds are considered more active and immediate in their effects, the root slower and deeper.

**Scientific:** All parts of the plant have shown broad-spectrum activity in scientific studies. The root has shown in vitro activity as an antibacterial agent against many pathogenic bacteria, an antiviral agent against HIV-1, an inhibitor of reverse transcriptase activity, a promoter of radical scavenging, an exceptionally strong antioxidant, and an antimutagenic agent. In vivo studies show antitumor and antitoxic activity (protecting from amaranth poisoning), antihepatotoxic activity (protecting the liver from $CCl_4$-induced hepatotoxicity), and anti-inflammatory activity (reducing various types of edema). Human trials have shown it to have antihyperglycemic activity, antitumor activity (delaying the progress of cancer), and hair-stimulant activity. The seeds have strong and specific antioxidant activity against LDLs.

## Preparation and Dosage

As tea, powder, capsules, tincture, or food.

**Root Preparations**

**Tea:** 1 tsp (5 mL) ground root per cup (8 ounces; 240 mL) water. Let steep in just-boiled water for 15–20 minutes. Drink 3 times per day.

**Powder:** 1–2 tsp (5–10 mL) up to 3 times per day.

**Capsules:** 2–4 "00" capsules 3 times a day.

**Tincture:** Many people prefer the fresh root. *Fresh,* 1:2 in 95 percent alcohol. *Dried,* 1:5 in 50 percent alcohol. 30–60 drops 3 times a day.

**Food:** The root can be added to stir-fry or boiled and eaten like parsnips. The stems can be peeled and cooked like okra in soups and stews.

**Seed Preparation**

**Tincture:** 1:5 in 60 percent alcohol, 5–25 drops up to 3 times per day.

### Contraindications and Side Effects

Contraindicated in patients with obstructed bile duct. Burdock may rarely cause contact dermatitis. A few people note headaches when taking the herb. If headache occurs, cease intake. No other side effects have been noted, although severe symptoms of anticholinergic-type poisoning were reported in a 26-year-old woman drinking "burdock" tea. A sample of the dried plant the woman had used for tea contained 30 percent atropine. Because atropine does not occur in burdock, the sample is generally recognized to have been adulterated; the correct identification of the plant is highly questionable. In addition, burdock has been used for millennia, and this is the only toxicity ever reported for the plant. It is highly unlikely that the herb in question was actually burdock.

## DANDELION *(Taraxacum officinale)*

**Family:** Compositae.
**Part used:** Whole plant.
**Collection and habitat:** Originally an Asian plant, it has traveled and settled everywhere. It may be harvested any time of the year. The leaves become more bitter with the season. As an additive to the diet, the leaves are usually picked in the spring until they flower. The flower is also deliciously edible and is used along with the leaves. Both are often used in salads. The root can be gathered at any time of the year. It is usually larger in the spring, before the plant sends up its leaves. Some evidence suggests that the fresh fall roots make the best tincture (although some people prefer the fresh spring roots). The fall roots have been found to be higher in inulin, one of dandelion's active constituents: 24 percent in October compared to 1.74 percent in March. If the plant is gathered while flowering and is hung up to dry, the flowers will quickly go to seed and your house will be covered with dandelion fluff.
**Actions:** *Leaves* — diuretic, nutritive, tonic, gastric secretion stimulant. *Root* — liver tonic, cholagogue, mild laxative.
**Functions in liver disease:** *Root* — hepatotonic, anti-inflammatory (reduces bile duct and liver inflammation), cholagogue. *Leaves* — diuretic, digestive bitter, mild cholagogue, and liver tonic. Reduces the

pressure on the liver to eliminate toxins by shunting more of the work to the kidneys.

**Specific indications:** *Root* — chronic liver disease, bile insufficiency, high bilirubin levels. *Leaves* — bile insufficiency, ascites.

## Uses of Dandelion

Dandelion is a very slow-acting herb. This makes it very good for hepatitis, which is a slowly progressive disease that develops over decades. Since dandelion is a food herb, it can be consumed in large quantities over long periods of time. The herb takes weeks to months to really begin showing its effects. It is one of the best supportive herbs for the liver; however, it does need other herbs that are more specific and energetic in their effects (such as bupleurum, phyllanthus, or turmeric) for complete success in healing hepatitis. It has been used in every culture in which it grows as a general tonic, liver, and blood herb as well as a food staple. According to the U.S. Department of Agriculture, 8 ounces (250 g) of raw dandelion greens contain 14,000 IU of vitamin A, compared to only 11,000 IU in raw carrots and 8100 IU in spinach. It is generally recommended that people consume 25,000 IU of vitamin A daily. Dandelion is also high in acetylcholine and chlorophyll.

**Ayurvedic:** Hepatotonic and stimulant, diaphoretic, cholagogue. Used in Ayurvedic practice for chronic liver disease, obstruction of the liver, jaundice, hepatitis, chronic skin disorders, and dyspepsia.

**Chinese:** In traditional Chinese medicine, dandelion is called "pu gong ying" and is thought to be specific for the liver and stomach. It is considered a cold herb, useful for hot conditions of the liver and stomach, such as hepatitis and ulceration (for which it has traditionally been used). It is believed to have the ability to reduce inflammation, dissipate heat, and detoxify the body. Chinese dosages are from 0.3 to 1.1 ounces (9–31 g) of whole dried plant consumed as a strong infusion in hot water daily.

**Western botanic practice:** Dandelion has come in and out of favor in western botanic practice as a tonic herb for the liver and as a diuretic. Nicholas Culpepper, the great English herbalist of the 17th century, found it useful in almost the same manner as conventional herbalists do today: "It is of an opening and cleansing quality, and therefore very effectual for the obstructions of the liver, gall, and spleen, and the diseases that arise from them, as the jaundice and hypochondriac."

**Scientific:** Oddly, most human dandelion trials were conducted early in this century; scientific circles in China and Japan seem to have little interest. A 1938 Italian trial explored the use of dandelion in people with liver dysfunction, jaundice, and low energy. Five mL of dandelion extract was injected daily for 20 days. Cholesterol and bilirubin levels were measured before and after this period. All participants but one showed significant cholesterol decrease and relief of jaundice; all reported higher energy levels. A 1950 human trial in England showed that dandelion was beneficial in hepatitis, jaundice, and liver enlargement. German clinical studies in the 1950s reported that an over-the-counter dandelion-centered preparation (Hepatichol) was associated with a significant improvement in cases of jaundice, acute and chronic bile duct inflammation, and gallbladder inflammation. The preparation also enhanced the concentration and secretion of bilirubin in the duodenum.

> ## Word Origin
>
> "Hypochondriac" originally was used to refer to people suffering from diseases of the liver; the hypochondrium is the part of the body where the liver is located.

In vivo, dandelion has been found to protect the liver from $CCl_4$-induced hepatotoxicity; to have antitumor and cytotoxic actions, choleretic activity, antihypercholesterolemic activity (reducing cholesterol in the blood), diuretic activity, and hypoglycemic action; and to be antispasmodic, anti-inflammatory (reducing chemically induced ear inflammation and carrageenan-induced pedal edema in mice), analgesic, and antiulcer. In vivo studies have also shown that dandelion stimulates bile flow to the same degree that injections of bile into the liver do. Other studies have indicated that this bile stimulation effect is an increase of three to four times normal.

## Preparation and Dosage

As a tea, tincture, powder, capsules, or food.

**Root Preparations**

**Tincture:** Fresh root (preferred), 1:2 in 95 percent alcohol. Dried root, 1:5 in 50 percent alcohol. ½–1 tsp (2.5–5 mL) per day.

**Tea:** ¼ ounce (8 g) cut and sifted root to 8 ounces (240 mL) water, boil slowly for 10 minutes, strain, cool, and drink. Up to 2 cups per day.

**Capsules:** 6–12 "00" capsules per day.

**Powder:** 2–6 tsp (10–30 mL) up to 3 times per day.

**Food:** Use like carrots.

**Leaf Preparations**

   **Tincture**: Fresh plant only, 1:2 in 95 percent alcohol. ½–2 tsp (2.5–10 mL) per day.

   **Tea:** 1 tsp (5 mL) dried herb to 8 ounces (240 mL) hot water. Steep 20 minutes. Drink as much as desired throughout the day.

   **Food:** In salads, use generous amounts and use often.

## Contraindications and Side Effects

Do not use in cases of bile duct obstruction. One common name for dandelion is piss-the-bed. If you are of middle age and have a typical aging bladder, do not stray far from bathroom facilities if you are taking much of the leaf, especially as a tea.

## MILK THISTLE (*Silybum marianum*)

**Family:** Asteraceae.

**Part used:** The seeds, especially the seed-vessel and pericarpium, although all parts of the plant may be used.

**Collection and habitat:** Considered a noxious weed, milk thistle prefers disturbed ground. Harvest when the heads have finished flowering and are showing puffy white fuzz that look a bit like parachutes.

**Actions:** Hepatoregenerator, hepatoprotective, hepatotonic, antihepatotoxic, choleretic, anticholestatic, anti-inflammatory for both liver and spleen, immunostimulant.

**Functions in liver disease:** Protecting the liver from the deleterious effects of hepatitis viruses; regenerating damaged liver tissue; tonifying, restoring, and normalizing liver function; reducing liver and spleen inflammation; stimulating bile production and flow; supporting immune function.

**Specific indications:** Cirrhosis or severe liver impairment, acute or chronic hepatitis, elevated liver enzyme levels, bile insufficiency, liver or spleen inflammation, feelings of abdominal pressure, fatigue, poor appetite.

## Uses of Milk Thistle

Milk thistle is one of the most potent herbs for protecting the liver against hepatotoxins and helping damaged liver tissue to regenerate. It is also the most extensively studied in clinical trials. The major active constituent is believed to be silymarin, which is found only in the seed and pericarpium. "Silymarin" is actually a combination name for three separate constituents of the herb. Milk thistle is also high in many other constituents, including betane, the primary constituent of beets. The herb is specifically for liver protection and regeneration and the normalization of liver function test results; it is not actively antiviral.

**Ayurvedic:** Not well known or used but historically present. Primarily used as a cholagogue.

**Chinese:** Milk thistle was unknown to TCM until introduced through modern research in Germany. Some TCM practitioners in China and abroad now commonly incorporate it into their treatment protocols for severe liver disease.

**Western botanic practice:** Milk thistle is western herbal medicine's primary contribution to the treatment of acute liver disease. The herb was well recognized at least 2000 years ago for its efficacy in promoting bile flow, relieving hepatic stagnation, and, in folk use, treating mushroom poisoning. Formerly called *Cardus marianum,* it enjoyed a resurgence in the 18th and 19th centuries when it was considered specific for spleen and liver inflammation and disease. Its popularity then faded and surged again through the research of German botanico-physicians in the 1960s. The research done since then firmly supports milk thistle as one of the most important herbs in the treatment of acute liver disease.

**Scientific:** Milk thistle and one of its constituents, silymarin, have been extensively tested in human trials for many years. Human trials have followed as few as 6 patients to as many as 2000 for up to 4 years.  The trials found that in cases of chronic alcoholic liver disease, toxic liver damage, type II hyperlipidemia, and steatorrhea, immune function was enhanced (T-cell and CD8 counts were raised); symptoms of tiredness, abdominal pressure, poor appetite, nausea, and itching were relieved; superoxide dismutase activity of white and red blood cells increased; liver function significantly improved; total cholesterol levels decreased; aminotransferase levels normalized; sulfobromophthalein sodium was retained; alanine aminotransferase and aspartate amino-transferase levels decreased or normalized; serum total and conju-gated bilirubin levels decreased; gamma-glutamyltransferase and leukocyte alkaline phosphatase values returned to normal; triglyc-eride levels declined markedly; and inflammation and toxic-meta-bolic lesions that had been verified through biopsy improved.

Several clinical trials have focused on hepatitis and cirrhosis. In hepatitis B trials, hepatic dysfunction markedly improved and HBsAg disappeared after treatment. Three studies of acute hepatitis found the following: shortened treatment time, as determined by alanine amino-transferase levels; improvement of serum levels of bilirubin, alanine aminotransferase, and aspartate aminotransferase; and much faster normalization of biochemical values than with placebo. Nine studies focusing on chronic hepatitis found significant improvement in patient population; normalization of liver function (as determined by biopsy); and relief of bloating, abdominal pressure, weakness, nervous-ness, and insomnia. The average time for improvements to be seen was 30 to 40 days.

In 11 studies focusing on cirrhosis, use of milk thistle was associ-ated with lower mortality rates; significant improvement in liver function test results (especially alanine aminotransferase, aspartate aminotransferase, and serum bilirubin levels); regression of inflam-matory changes and regression of toxic-metabolic lesions; significant improvement in liver cell permeability, metabolic efficiency, and excretory function; and alleviation of symptoms such as bloating, insomnia, abdominal pressure, and increased body weight. Perhaps the most impres-sive studies of the actions of milk this-tle have been in cases of poisoning with *Amanita phalloides* mushrooms. These mushrooms contain one of the most potent liver toxins known — phal-loidin. Several interventions in poison-ing cases in Germany found that milk thistle protected the liver from the action of the toxin and reversed liver damage. Optimum results occurred

## Milk Thistle Seeds

Milk thistle seeds may be pre-pared like pumpkin seeds and are quite tasty. Lightly toast them in a hot frying pan, salt with tamari or soy, and eat as desired throughout the day. The leaves of the plant (with the spines cut away) may be eaten in salads, and the root may be roasted or boiled.

when the poisoning cases were treated within 48 hours. Mortality rates were reduced from 50 percent to 10 percent.

Both in vivo and in vitro studies have shown similar results. In addition, milk thistle has shown consistent choleretic, antibacterial, and anticholestatic activity.

### Preparation and Dosage

As tincture, capsules, powder, or food. Many experts feel that the active constituent of milk thistle is poorly water soluble, precluding milk thistle's use as a tea. It is often suggested that the seeds be prepared as a standardized alcohol extract to provide the greatest benefit. Many practitioners believe that the whole herb and a nonstandardized tincture work as well.

**Standardized tincture (store-bought):** Standardized to 80 mg silybum flavonoids (40 drops 3 times per day for 6–9 months) or 140 mg silybum flavonoids (25 drops 3 times per day for 6–9 months).

**Tincture (powdered seed):** 1:3 in 70 percent alcohol; ½–1 tsp (2.5–5 mL) up to 4 times per day for 6–9 months.

**Capsules and powder:** For acute or chronic hepatitis, from 4 "00" capsules of powdered seed 3 times per day up to 3 tbl (45 mL) of the powdered seed per day for 6–9 months.

### Contraindications and Side Effects

None noted.

## PHYLLANTHUS *(Phyllanthus niruri, P. amarus, P. emblica)*

**Family:** Euphorbiacae.

**Part used:** All parts of the plant and the fruit of *P. emblica.* With *P. niruri* and *P. amarus,* the dried plant was used in human trials. With *P. emblica,* the dried fruit was used.

**Collection and habitat:** There is some disagreement among herbalists regarding the inclusion of *P. emblica* under a general "phyllanthus" listing. It possesses two Latin names *(P. emblica* and *Emblica officinalis)* that I have found to be synonymous in nearly every reference guide. Some books list it under one name, some the other. It, along with the two other *Phyllanthus* species listed here, is a member of the Euphorbiaceae family. However, it grows as a substantial perennial shrub to large tree. It is native to tropical Asia and grows in mixed hardwood forests. Although all parts of the plant are used, the fruits are especially prized and contain 20 times more vitamin C than orange juice does. *P. emblica* is one of the main ingredients of the famous Ayurvedic triphala formula, which also contains two other plants, both *Terminalia* species. In contrast, both *P. amarus* and *P. niruri* are short, shrubby, annual herbs that grow to 2 feet tall and are common across the tropics in Africa and Asia.

The fruits of *P. emblica* are harvested when ripe; the whole plants of *P. niruri* and *P. amarus* are harvested when they are in flower. Both fruit and plants are generally used dried rather than fresh.

**Actions:** Anti-inflammatory, hepatoprotective, antiviral, antihepatotoxic, hepatic tonic, diuretic, astringent, antifungal.

**Functions in liver disease:** Antiviral — specific against hepatitis viruses, especially HBV (inactivates HBsAg, inhibits HBsAg expression); protects liver against liver disease/chemical toxins; serves as a tonic for the liver; alleviates skin problems associated with hepatitis; helps excretion by helping the kidneys take some of the load off the liver; reduces liver inflammation.

**Specific indications:** Viral hepatitis, portal inflammation, elevated liver enzyme levels, poor appetite, skin eruptions associated with liver disease.

## Uses of Phyllanthus

Phyllanthus has been brought to the attention of western herbalism through Ayurvedic practice. Most of the studies have been conducted in India, with a handful from the United States, England, Australia, and China. Pyllanthus can be a rather difficult herb to find; some sources are listed in the appendix.

**Ayurvedic:** *P. niruri* is called "bhumy amalaki" in traditional Ayurvedic practice. It clears liver obstruction and is an alterative, diuretic, and astringent; it is cooling to hot conditions. Used for jaundice, chronic dysentery, and cirrhosis of the liver. *P. emblica* is also known as *E. officinalis* and is called "amala" or "amalak" or (sometimes) "emblic myrobalan" in Ayurvedic practice. It is considered to have actions similar to those of *P. niruri* and is also refrigerant, laxative, carminative, and stomachic.

**Chinese:** Apparently unknown.

**Western botanic practice:** Two *Phyllanthus* species grow in the western hemisphere: 1) *P. liebmannianus,* which is used in South America in indigenous practice for stomatitis, internal infections, kidney stones, and stoppage of urine; and 2) *P. caroliniensis,* which grows in the United States as far west as Texas and as far north as Ohio. Despite this, the use of phyllanthus in western herbal practice has been uncommon. Ayurvedic practice has introduced its modern use as a hepatic tonic and antiviral for hepatitis. Given the broad activity of phyllanthus against hepatitis viruses, it seems likely that these two western species will also prove beneficial.

**Scientific:** Fourteen species of phyllanthus have been tested for activity against hepatitis viruses and found to be active in vivo, in vitro, or in human trials. The primary varieties tested in humans are *P. amarus* and *P. niruri.* In general, these are considered the most reliably active phyllanthus species for treatment of hepatitis.

*P. amarus:* Eight trials noted. Both dried encapsulated plant powder and tea/infusions were used in the trials for treatment of HBV infection. Three trials reported that 60 percent of patients went from being HBsAg positive to being HBsAg negative. Two clinical trials of patients with chronic hepatitis (non-A, non-B) noted decreased plasma bilirubin levels, improvement of sulfobromophthalein sodium clearance, and marked attenuation of portal inflammation. Two trials of acute viral hepatitis found that liver function significantly improved in both HBsAg-negative and HBsAg-positive patients. One double-blind clinical trial of patients with hepatitis B reported that 50 percent of those who received *P. amarus* compared with 4 percent of patients who received placebo cleared HBsAg by the first return visit.

*P. niruri:* Two trials noted. In one, children with acute viral hepatitis were treated by *P. niruri* extract; liver function returned to normal within 5 days. A second trial found that in children with infective hepatitis, appetite normalized within 5 weeks.

All tested phyllanthus species showed antiviral activity against many viruses (primarily hepatitis viruses) and hepatoprotective activity against a variety of chemical toxins in vitro and in vivo.

*One note:* The hepatitis trials used, on average, 600 mg of *P. amarus* herb per day or, in one case, 200 mg as a strong infusion once per day. *P. emblica* dosage in a human trial was included in a multiple herb mixture and consisted of 500 mg per person per day for all herbs. That trial was a double-blind study of a multicomponent mix for people with acute viral hepatitis. It also contained *Terminalia chebula, T. belerica, Commiphora mukul, Plumbago Zeylanica,* and *Picrorhiza kurroa.*

## Preparation and Dosage

As tea or powder or in capsules.

**P. niruri and P. amarus Preparations**
  **Tea:** 1 tsp (5 mL) infusion of plant in 8 ounces (240 mL) water 2 times per day.
  **Powder:** 1 tsp (5 mL) powdered leaf up to 2 times per day (5–6 g up to 3 times per day) in water or juice.
  **Capsules:** 2–4 "00" capsules up to 3 times per day.

**P. emblica and E. officinalis Preparations**
**Powder of dried fruit:** 2–3 tsp (10–20 g) in water or juice, 3–4 times per day.

> ### Dosage Note
>
> Ayurvedic dosage for jaundice is 1 tsp (5 mL) powdered leaf of *P. niruri* in 8 ounces (240 mL) water 2 times per day. *P. amarus* can be found as standardized capsules under the trade name Phyllanthol (see Resources).

## Contraindications and Side Effects

None noted.

## PICRORHIZA *(Picrorhiza kurroa)*

**Family:** Scrophulariaceae.
**Part used:** Generally the root, although the whole plant has been found to be active and is sometimes used in traditional practice.
**Collection and habitat:** Picrorhiza is a common plant in the northwestern Himalayas, and the pencil-thin roots are harvested in the fall or at any time needed.
**Actions:** Hepatotonic, antiviral, antiperiodic, bitter tonic, cholagogue, immunostimulant, alterative, stomachic, antipyretic, laxative, antiasthmatic (inhibiting bronchial constriction response, inhibiting histamine release, increasing bronchial dilation), antiprotozoal, antiparasitic, and antidysenteric.

**Functions in liver disease:** Antiviral against hepatitis viruses, protects liver from damage by hepatitis, normalizes liver function and liver enzyme levels, combats recurrent fever and chills, enhances immune function, stimulates digestive and pancreatic insulin secretion, aids the liver in converting sugar to glycogen and storing it for future use.

**Specific indications:** Viral hepatitis, elevated liver enzyme levels, liver damage or cirrhosis, intermittent fever and chills, reduced liver function.

## Uses of Picrorhiza

Picrorhiza is the least well known of the Ayurvedic herbs for treatment of hepatitis; most research on it has been done in India. Many trials have used a standardized extract: picroliv (sometimes available in the United States; see Resources). However, at least three other constituents (and the whole herb) have been found to be active for liver disease in separate studies. Ayurvedic clinicians report excellent success with the herb in clinical practice in treatment of HAV, HBV, and HCV infections. Generally, they have found liver enzyme levels to return to normal within 7 days among patients with HAV infection and in 3 weeks to 3 months for patients with HBV and HCV infections. The herb is exceptionally bitter to the taste.

**Ayurvedic:** In India, picrorhiza is also called "katuka," "katula," or "kutki," not to be confused with "kala kutki" (black hellebore). It is considered to be a bitter tonic that is as efficacious as gentian and is a hepatotonic, antiasthmatic, pneumatic, and antidysenteric agent. Picrorhiza has been used for giardiasis, amebiasis, and liver and autoimmune diseases. It is often used as an antiperiodic in returning conditions of alternating fever and chills, such as malaria, elephantiasis, and ill-defined feverish conditions.

**Chinese:** Used in China and Korea but not well known. Rare in TCM.

**Western botanic practice:** Generally unknown in western practice until its recent introduction in the treatment of hepatitis.

**Scientific:** Picrorhiza and various of its constituents have been found to be significantly active in human trials and in double-blind studies of hepatitis viruses (2 g per day orally) both alone and in combination with other herbs, such as phyllanthus (500 mg oral combination dosage). In vivo studies have found picrorhiza and its constituents to be broadly antihepatotoxic and hepatoprotective against many potent hepatotoxins; it specifically protects against hepatotoxicity caused by thioacetamide, $CCl_4$, galactosamine, rifampicin, paracetamol, ethanol/ $CCl_4$, aflatoxin B1, *Amanita phalloides*, monocrotaline, and *Plasmodium bergheri* (a potent liver parasite). In all instances, liver function improved dramatically; for example, in cases of monocrotaline-induced hepatotoxicity, levels of hepatic succinate dehydrogenase, acid ribonuclease, acid phosphatase, gamma-glutamyl transpeptidase, 5'-nucleotidase, glucose-6-phosphatase, cytochrome P450 activity, glycogen, albumin, and protein all increased. DNA repair was enhanced, and serum bilirubin levels decreased. In galactosamine- and paracetamol-induced liver damage, serum alanine aminotransferase, aspartate aminotransferase, acid phosphatase, alkaline phosphatase, glutamate dehydrogenase, and bilirubin levels decreased.

The standardized extract, picroliv, caused significant reversal in all affected enzymes in both galactosamine- and thioacetamide-induced liver damage. It also reversed decreased incorporation of leucine into liver protein. In aflatoxin B1 liver damage, treated animals showed improvement of hepatocyte alteration in liver lobules and portal tract and of liver enzyme production and macromolecule synthesis. Use of the whole herb reversed the decrease in liver function caused by partial removal of the liver. Pretreatment with picrorhiza for 15 days prevented $CCl_4$ damage to the liver. Picrorhiza, alpha lipoic acid, and milk thistle seed (and possibly reishi) are the only substances I am aware of that can counter the potent toxins in *Amanita phalloides* mushrooms.

## Preparation and Dosage

The tincture is sometimes used (1:5 in 60 percent alcohol; ¼ tsp [1.25 mL] 2–3 times per day), but it is exceptionally bitter and difficult to take. The general and preferred form of consumption is the powdered herb in capsules: 1–3 g (that is, 2–6 "00" capsules) 2–3 times per day. Sometimes the powdered herb is given in juice, 1 tsp (5 mL) up to 2 times per day.

## Contraindications and Side Effects

Contraindicated in patients with obstructed bile duct. Larger doses may be emetic and purgative. If nausea or diarrhea occurs, reduce the dosage or take with food. Some people have reported skin rash.

## REISHI *(Ganoderma lucidum)*

**Family:** Ganodermataceae.

**Part used:** Generally the fruiting body (that is, the mushroom itself); sometimes the mycelium.

**Collection and habitat:** At any time. The fungus grows on trees throughout the world.

**Actions:** Antiviral (against numerous viruses, including HBV and HIV), hepatoregenerator, antihepatotoxic, choleretic, hypocholesterolemic, antihyperbilirubinemic, antihyperlipidemic, antihypertriglyceridemic, cholagogue, immunomodulator, immunostimulant (stimulates interleukin-1 and -2, phagocytosis, lymphocyte proliferation, and interferon-gamma production; enhances natural killer cells; activates macrophages; enhances polymorphonuclear leukocytes; protects and enhances T cells; enhances thymus weight and functioning; stimulates interferon-gamma production), antitumor (reduces proliferation of tumor cells and inhibits tumor-necrosis factor), cytotoxic, antibacterial, hypotensive, antinephrotoxic, antiallergenic, spleen and thymus tonic, coronary vasodilator, analgesic, anti-inflammatory.

**Functions in liver disease:** Lessens liver pain, enhances weight gain, normalizes liver enzyme levels, protects against cirrhosis, reduces collagen content in liver cirrhosis, inhibits lipid peroxide formation, increases mental clarity, serves as a hepatoprotective agent, has antiviral actions against HBV and probably HCV, helps resolve sleep disorders, reduces dizziness, acts as a broadly active immunostimulant, has immunomodulator actions, and reduces cholesterol levels.

**Specific indications**: Chronic viral infection, liver pain, brain fog, sleep disorder, liver damage or cirrhosis, elevated liver enzyme levels, weight loss, depleted immune function, liver cancer, portal hypertension.

### Uses of Reishi

Reishi is a hard, woody, reddish-capped mushroom that usually grows on trees. It is well known in Asia and is only recently becoming recognized in western botanic and medical practice.

**Ayurvedic:** Apparently unknown.

**Chinese:** Ganoderma is known as "ling zhi" in China and "reishi" in Japan. It is now commonly known as reishi in the west. Reishi has been used in China and Japan for at least 4000 years in the treatment of hepatitis, kidney disease, arthritis, hypertension, sleep disorders, asthma and bronchitis, ulcer, and nerve pain. In TCM, it is considered warming, tonic, nourishing, antitoxic, and astringent and is thought to disperse accumulations. At least five species of *Ganoderma* are used in traditional medicine in China and Japan, each for different disorders. In many respects, *G. lucidum* is considered the most potent.

**Western botanic practice:** Apparently unknown until its introduction by traditional Chinese practitioners. Western use has been stimulated by the extensive studies conducted in Japan.

**Scientific:** In vivo and in vitro studies have found reishi to normalize liver enzyme levels; to be liver regenerative, liver protective, choleretic, analgesic, antiallergenic, anti-inflammatory, antibacterial, antiviral, antioxidant, antitumor (inhibiting or regressing tumors), hypotensive, cardiotonic, expectorant, and antitussive; and to serve as a bronchial relaxant and immunostimulant.

Human trials have found effectiveness for neurasthenia, insomnia, dizziness, duodenal ulcers, liver pain, rhinitis, muscular dystrophy, stress, Alzheimer's disease, hyperlipidemia, liver failure, diabetes, and hepatitis.

In one human trial of 355 people with hepatitis B receiving a combination formula containing reishi, 92.4 percent of patients showed improvement. Another trial found that in patients with hepatitis B, hepatitis symptoms were alleviated and aminotransferase levels decreased. Other trials showed reduction in blood pressure in all hypertensive patients who took reishi for 6 months. In trials with over 2000 patients with chronic bronchitis, 60 to 90 percent of patients experienced alleviation of symptoms, marked improvement in overall health, and weight gain. Studies of people with high blood pressure have consistently shown decreases in blood pressure, and studies among people with impaired memory or thinking have shown improved mental clarity and memory. Reishi has a long history of folk and historical clinical use in protecting the liver against *Amanita phalloides* poisoning, although I could locate no specific trials.

The studies are fairly extensive; a broad sampling can be found in the references or in Christopher Hobbs' excellent book *Medicinal Mushrooms* (Interweave Press, 1996). It is clear that reishi is one of the most potent herbal medicines for treatment of hepatitis and liver disease.

## Preparation and Dosage

May be taken as soup, powder, syrup decoction, tablets, or tincture.

**Tablets (store-bought):** Three 1 g tablets, 3 times per day.

**Tincture:** (1:5 in 20 percent alcohol) 2–4 tsp (10–20 mL) 3 times per day.

**Syrup decoction:** Use 2–5 g reishi per quart (L) of water depending on strength desired. Slowly bring to boil and simmer at lowest boil obtainable for 2 hours, uncovered, until the volume of water is reduced by two-thirds. Cool and strain. Consume in the evening before bed or in three equal amounts over the course of the day. For acute conditions, the amount consumed can be increased as much as desired.

**Powder:** 3–6 g per day for chronic disease, 9–15 g per day for acute conditions. Divide into 3 equal doses. Stir into water and drink or encapsulate (6–12 "00" capsules for chronic disease, 18–30 capsules for acute conditions). For mushroom poisoning, 120–200 g dried powdered reishi in water, 3–5 times per day.

## Contraindications and Side Effects

Contraindicated in obstructed bile duct. Skin rash, loose stool, dry mouth, and nausea sometimes occur. Adverse reactions cease upon discontinuation of reishi use. If nausea occurs, consume reishi with meals.

# TURMERIC *(Curcuma longa)*

**Family:** Zingiberaceae.

**Part used:** Usually the root, although the leaf and oleoresin may sometimes be used.

**Collection and habitat:** Generally commercially grown in India and Asia. The roots are harvested in late fall or early winter. The roots are washed, well boiled, and dried in the sun. They may then be powdered for commercial culinary turmeric or thinly sliced for later use as herbal medicine.

**Actions:** Antiviral, antihepatotoxic, anticholesterolemic, cholagogue, cholestatic, choletonic, cholecystokinetic, immunostimulant (stimulates interferon production, increases phagocytosis), antioxidant, antiinflammatory, antitumor, cytotoxic, antibacterial, antiparasitic, blood refrigerant, inhibitory of platelet aggregation factor.

**Functions in liver disease:** Acts as anti-inflammatory, protects against lipid peroxide formation, promotes production and flow of bile, protects against and reverses liver damage, reduces cholesterol and LDL levels, increases HDL levels, removes excess accumulation of cholesterol in the liver, increases conversion of cholesterol into bile acids, protects against formation of and retards liver cancer, has immunostimulatory actions, potentiates adrenal hormone activity, and serves as an antioxidant. Relieves the arthritis, dyspepsia, skin conditions, and allergy symptoms that often accompany liver disease.

**Specific indications:** Liver damage, liver cancer, cirrhosis, elevated cholesterol levels, decreased bile production and flow, insufficient bile salts. Liver disease–associated arthritis, skin eruptions, asthma, and bronchitis.

## Uses of Turmeric

Turmeric, which is primarily known as a spice (it gives curry its well-known yellow color), is gaining recognition among western clinical practitioners as one of the most potent liver herbs (along with milk thistle, reishi, bupleurum, and phyllanthus) for the treatment of hepatitis.

**Ayurvedic:** Turmeric is commonly known as "besar" or "haldi." Nine types of turmeric are grown throughout India, of which *Curcuma longa* is the most popularly cultivated. In Ayurvedic and Unani practice, it is used for intermittent fevers; for removal of liver obstruction; and for jaundice, dropsy, impurity of the blood, and skin conditions, such as eczema and psoriasis.

**Chinese:** Known in China as "jiang huang," turmeric and another turmeric species, *C. aromatica* or wild turmeric (yu jin), are both used extensively in Chinese medicine. Turmeric has been used since the 7th century, probably entering Chinese practice from India. It is official in the Chinese pharmacopeia and is used to remove blood stasis, promote and normalize energy flow in the body, and relieve pain. It is considered to have specific affinity for the liver and spleen.

**Western botanic practice:** Unknown until recently except as a spice.

**Scientific:** Turmeric has been extensively explored in the past several years in several studies in Korea, Japan, India, China, and Indonesia. In vitro studies have shown it to have specific activity against HBV and HIV-1 and to be antihepatotoxic, protecting against aceta-minophen- and $CCl_4$-induced liver damage. In vivo studies have shown liver protective activity against liver disease induced by afla-toxin B1, acetaminophen, $CCl_4$, alpha-naphthylisothicyanate, and beta-D-galactosamine. Further studies showed consistent choleretic activity (in one instance increasing bile acid output by nearly 100 percent), anticomplement and antihypercholesterolemic activity, and antihyperlipidemic activity.

Other in vivo studies with one active constituent of turmeric — curcumin — have shown that it decreases cholesterol and LDL levels and increases HDL levels. Furthermore, curcumin and turmeric both decrease levels of lipid peroxidation and reverse liver damage in vivo. Curcumin also reduces the production of cholesterol gallstones.

Human trials with turmeric have shown that the herb is effective as an antiasthmatic (for chronic bronchitis or asthma), an anti-inflammatory (for osteoarthritis), and an antidyspeptic. The latter two trials were randomized, double-blind studies. Trials of curcumin use in humans have shown that it decreases levels of serum lipid per-oxides, increases HDL levels, and decreases total serum cholesterol levels.

Several other in vitro studies have shown consistent antimycobac-terial (antituberculous) activity and cytotoxic, antioxidant, antibac-terial, antifungal, antiviral, antimutagenic, and platelet aggregation inhibition actions.

Many in vivo studies have reported carcinogenesis inhibition, antitumor activity, protection against the DNA damage associated with cancer formation, immunostimulant activity, interferon stimu-lation, increases in phagocytosis, anti-inflammatory activity against various induced edemas, antimutagenic action, general antitoxic activity, antiulcer activity, anticoagulant action, and wound-healing acceleration. Commercial-grade turmeric prevented the formation of cancer in mice (liver, forestomach, duodenum, and colon) and reduced tumor size in mice with cancer. It has been found to be active against cancer in various parts, including the liver, of numerous species of laboratory animals.

## Preparation and Dosage

Because of the quantities necessary, turmeric is most easily used in herbal medicine as a paste or a powder blended in juice or water. Some practitioners recommend an extract standardized for curcumin content. These extracts are commonly found in health food stores. Turmeric may also be used as a tincture, in capsules, or in food.

**Paste:** Make into turmeric paste and roll into marble-sized, pill-like balls. Put in back of throat, and swallow with lots of water. Take 4 per day for acute or chronic hepatitis.

**Powder:** 1 tsp (5 mL) powder blended into water or juice up to 4 times per day.

**Tincture:** Dry powdered root: 1:5 in 50 percent alcohol, 10–30 drops 3 times per day.

**Capsules:** As tonic, 2–6 "00" capsules up to 3 times per day.

**Food:** Consume tumeric often in food and use generously.

## Contraindications and Side Effects

Do not use if there is bile obstruction. Turmeric is brilliantly yellow and may stain hands, clothes, and utensils.

## Turmeric Paste

*Here is a great way to prepare turmeric for use in liver disease. Usually people use 1–3 marble-sized balls, lightly rolled between the fingers and swallowed with water.*

> ¼ cup (50 g) turmeric powder
> ½ cup (120 mL) water

Combine turmeric and water in a saucepan, bring to a low boil, and cook, stirring frequently, until mixture becomes a thick paste. Remove from heat and let cool. Store in refrigerator in sealed container.

## A FEW FINAL HERBS OF NOTE

Several other herbs and combinations of herbs have shown effectiveness against hepatitis viruses and liver cirrhosis in human trials. The trials for these herbs are listed in the reference section of the appendix.

• *Berberis aristata:* bark, 2 g per day per person, active against hepatitis, similar to barberry *(Berberis vulgaris).*

• *Polyporus umbellatus:* intramuscular injection of a polysaccharide fraction of the mushroom, dosed at 40 mg per day for 3 months. In 359 patients treated, symptoms and biochemical test results improved.

• *Carduus nutans:* leaf, alcohol tincture, dose not stated; active in human hepatitis trials.

• *Cochlospermum planchonii:* root, water infusion, dose not stated; comatose patients with sudden onset of hepatitis recovered. Biological activity was highly dose-dependent.

• *Cotinus coggygria:* branches and leaves, hot water decoction, dose not stated; 400 patients with hepatitis were treated, with a success rate of 94 percent.

• *Eclipta alba:* whole plant, dried, oral administration of 500 mg per person 3 times per day cured jaundice in 75 percent; same rate of cure was noted at lower dose (50 mg per person) in children with jaundice; plant has also been found to be strongly hepatoprotective and antihepatotoxic in vivo and in vitro.

• *Paeonia rubra:* dried root, hot water decoction, dose not stated; protected against and reversed cholestatic hepatitis.

• *Rheum officinale:* dried root, single dose of only 50 mg per person was found to be active in protecting the liver and healing in 80 cases of icteric hepatitis.

• *Sedum sarmentosum:* whole plant, dried, hot water decoction, dose not stated; found to be active in a double-blind, controlled trial of hot infusion in treatment of patients with hepatitis.

• *Symphytum officinale* a.k.a. comfrey: whole plant, dose not stated, purified wood vinegar obtained by carbonization of wood under semi-aerobic conditions was used as the extraction medium for the comfrey; extract was then repeatedly used to treat adults with liver cirrhosis and was found to be active for healing that condition.

- **Combination mixture** of *Gardenia jasminoides, Angelica sinensis, Atractylodes macrocephala, Paeonia albiflora, Salvia miltiorrhiza, Artemisia scoparia, Astragalus membranaceus, Rehmannia glutinosa, Paeonia moutan,* and *Poria cocos:* decoction, dose not stated; 105 patients with cirrhosis were treated for 2–18 months. Liver function and liver health were improved or restored to normal, and enlarged liver and spleen were reduced and softened. Sixty-seven patients recovered completely, 14 showed marked improvement, 17 showed some improvement, and 7 did not respond to treatment. After 12 months, relapse occurred in 13.4 percent.
- **Combination mixture** of *Achillea millefolium, Capparis spinosa, Cassia occidentalis, Cichorium intybus, Solanum nigrum, Tamarix gallica,* and *Terminalia arjuna:* hot water decoction, dose not stated; successful in treating hepatitis in human trials.
- **Combination mixture** of fresh leaf of *Citrus reticulata, Astragalus membranaceus, Smilax china, Gardenia jasminoides, Pueraria lobata, Curcuma aromatica, Glycyrrhiza glabra, Vigna sinensis:* hot water decoction, 6 tsp (30 mL) per person; 120 cases of hepatitis B (with a 48-person control group) were treated twice per day for 1–3 months (average, 60 days); in 72 patients, the virus was cleared and jaundice disappeared, and in 36, symptoms significantly improved.

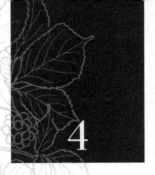

# BOTANICAL SUPPORT
# FOR THE IMMUNE SYSTEM

Research reported in the April 14, 2000, issue of the journal *Science* found that the health of the immune system is significantly related to the progress of HCV infection. The healthier the immune system, the smaller the variation in the HCV viral swarm. This limit on virus variability results in a less severe long-term disease. In addition, a healthier immune system helps lessen the fatigue that is often experienced as the body fights off the disease or a new variant of the virus, which can take energy away from the rest of the body. These two factors make it important that the immune system be supported throughout the course of HCV infection.

## QUALITIES OF IMMUNE-BOOSTING HERBS

In choosing immune herbs for treatment of hepatitis C, it is important to look for herbs that singly or together do three things: 1) stimulate and support the parts of the immune system that are most affected by the disease; 2) stimulate the parts of the immune system that most effectively help deactivate the disease; and 3) exert strong liver protective activity. Of particular importance are herbs that stimulate interferon and antibody production, herbs that support overall immune strength, herbs that reduce stress, and herbs that help improve energy levels.

## 10 Major Immune Tonic Herbs for Hepatitis

| | | |
|---|---|---|
| Ashwagandha | Licorice | Siberian ginseng |
| Astragalus | Panax ginseng | Tienchi ginseng |
| Boneset | Red root | |
| Codonopsis | Schizandra | |

## ASHWAGANDHA *(Withania somnifera)*

**Family:** Solanaceae.

**Part used:** The root is used in western practice, and all parts of the plant are used in the rest of the world.

**Collection and habitat:** The plant is little grown (or known) in North America but is common in India, the Sudan, Pakistan, Iraq, Saudi Arabia, and Rwanda. The root is usually harvested in the fall, the leaves can be harvested at any time, and the seeds are harvested in season.

**Actions:** *Root* — immune tonic, stress-protective, antihepatotoxic, antibacterial, diuretic, antipyretic, astringent, nerve sedative, alterative. *Leaves and stem* — antihepatotoxic, antipyretic, febrifuge, bitter, diuretic, antibacterial, antimicrobial, astringent, nerve sedative. *Seeds* — hypnotic, diuretic, coagulant. *Fruit (of related species)* — immune tonic, antibacterial, alterative.

**Functions in liver disease:** Antistressor, immune tonic and potentiator, antihepatotoxic; stimulates glutathione production, alleviates irritability and mental confusion, reduces joint pain.

### About Ashwagandha

Ashwagandha has a reputation as a strong and sure immune tonic and stress protector that rivals ginseng. It has a millennia-long tradition of use in northern Africa, India, and portions of Asia. One of its strengths is its reliable action as a nervine sedative. For people who are highly stressed, the herb gently lowers stress levels in the body, protects the body from stress-related disease, and brings the immune system up to optimum levels of activity.

In vivo studies have shown that ashwagandha possesses strong hepatoprotective and antihepatotoxic properties, protecting the liver from hepatotoxicity induced by $CCl_4$, rifampin, acetaminophen, and galactosamine and decreasing cadmium-induced lipid peroxidation. It also shows marked hypolipemic activity: the herb is associated with decreases in serum beta-lipoprotein, apoprotein, and LDL levels. Nonspecific resistance is increased (eosinophil counts increased during swimming endurance tests), stress endurance is extended, and phagocytosis increases. Other in vivo studies have shown that ashwagandha is anti-inflammatory (reducing various edemas), antileukopenic, antitoxic, antitumor, antiulcer, anticonvulsant, a carcinogenesis inhibitor, and a stimulator of glutathione production.

In vitro studies have shown that ashwagandha possesses antibacterial, antiyeast, antifungal, antiamoebic, antimalarial, antiviral (against herpes simplex virus 1 and others), and immunostimulant (stimulating interferon induction) activity.

Human trials have tended to use ashwagandha combined with other herbs. One randomized, double-blind, crossover, placebo-controlled study in patients with osteoarthritis found significant alleviation of pain and stiffness, increases in grip strength, and reduction in disability score. Ashwagandha, turmeric, zinc, and *Boswellia serrata* were used. Another multicomponent trial found ashwagandha good for sexual dysfunction.

Of interest, in both animal and human studies ashwagandha has been found to have distinct effects on the brain: It acts as a central nervous system depressant (sedative), relieves psychosis (in combination with other herbs), and reduces aggression and stress levels.

Two other *Withania* species are used in much the same manner. *W. obtusifolia* has a long history of use in the Sudan, and *W. coagulans* (especially the fruit) has long been used in Pakistan and India. The latter herb is so termed because it is a powerful coagulating agent and Indians use it in place of rennet to make cheese.

## Preparation and Dosage

The herb is available almost exclusively through larger health food stores, although some bulk suppliers are beginning to carry it. Ashwagandha is usually prepared as capsules of the powdered root. Follow manufacturer directions or use 2 "00" capsules up to 3 times per day as a tonic. For chronic or acute liver disease, up to 2 tsp (10 mL) of the powdered root may be taken per day.

## Contraindications and Side Effects

Ashwagandha is used in India as an abortifacient. Not suggested for use during pregnancy.

## △ASTRAGALUS  *(Astragalus membranaceous)*

**Family:** Leguminosae.
**Part used:** The plant is a perennial with a long fibrous root stock. The root is used for medicine.
**Collection and habitat:** The plant grows in Asia and is primarily harvested in China; it has been used in Chinese medicine for millennia. The root is often found thinly sliced and dried, and it most closely resembles a yellow tongue depressor. The powdered root or coarsely ground organic root is also becoming increasingly available in the marketplace.
**Actions:** Immune system enhancer, stimulant, and restorative; antiviral; adaptogen; tonic; antihepatotoxic; diuretic; enhances function in lungs, spleen, and digestive tract.
**Function in liver disease:** Antiviral, immune stimulant and potentiator; stimulates antibody formation and interferon production; specifically stimulates the immune system to respond to viruses; has antihepatotoxic, antitumor, antimetastatic actions.

## About Astragalus

Astragalus has been found to be exceptionally effective for the immune system. Clinical studies have reported that astragalus protects the human heart from Coxsackie B2 virus and helps repair damage in previously infected people. Other studies have shown that astragalus enhances the body's own natural killer cell activity. As an antitumor agent, astragalus prevented cancer metastasis in 80 percent of mice tested. Still other studies have shown that astragalus stimulates T-cell activity and restores immune function in cancer patients with impaired immune function. Astragalus's action is comprehensive. Robyn Landis and K. P. Khalsa note that "astragalus stimulates phagocytosis (invader-engulfing activity), increasing the total number of cells and the aggressiveness of their activity. Increased macrophage activity has been measured as lasting up to seventy-two hours. It increases the number of stem cells (the 'generic' cells that can become any type needed) in the marrow and lymph tissue, stimulates their maturation into active immune cells, increases spleen activity, increases releases of antibodies, and boosts the production of hormonal messenger molecules that signal for virus destruction."

At the University of Texas Medical Center in Houston, researchers noted that astragalus could completely restore the function of cancer patients' compromised immune cells. Other human trials showed that astragalus increased serum immunoglobulin E, immunoglobulin M, and cyclic adenosine monophosphate and stimulated interferon induction and natural killer cell formation. Astragalus has also been found in human trials to be directly active against several viruses, including Coxsackie B and herpes (progenitalis).

In vivo studies have shown that astragalus has exceptional immune-stimulating action (interferon induction stimulation, enhanced antibody response, increased antibody formation, increased phagocytosis, stimulation of lymphocyte blastogenesis, stimulation of interleukin-6 formation and T lymphocytes) and action against a variety of viruses and cancers. Astragalus has also shown consistent antihepatotoxic activity against a variety of hepatotoxins, antihyperglycemic activity, and inhibition of aminotransferases.

Because of its antiviral, immunostimulant effects (especially in formation and enhancement of antibodies and stimulation of interleukin and interferon) and its hepatoprotective and antihepatotoxic actions, astragalus is a primary herb to use in the treatment of HCV infection.

## Preparations and Dosage

May be taken as tea, capsules, tincture, or powder or in food.

**Tea:** 2–3 ounces (60–180 mL) herb to pot of tea; drink throughout the day.

**Capsules:** 3 "00" capsules 3 times per day as immune tonic. For viral infections, 8 g per day (5–6 capsules 3 times per day).

**Tincture:** 1:5 in 60 percent alcohol, 30–60 drops up to 4 times per day.

**Powder:** For chronic or acute liver disease, up to 3 tbl (54 mL) per day may be consumed.

**Food:** Two of the best ways to use astragalus as food are as a broth base for soups and as a rice.

### Contraindications and Side Effects

No toxicity from the ingestion of astragalus has ever been shown. The Chinese report that the herb has been consistently used for millennia to treat colds and flu and suppressed immune function.

---

## Immune-Enhancing Rice

*Here is a great way to add immune power to rice. Use as you would any rice, as a base for meals throughout the week.*

>      4 cups water
>      2 cups brown rice
>      1½ ounces sliced astragalus root

**1.** Add astragalus to water, bring to boil, and simmer for 2 hours covered.

**2.** Remove from heat and let stand overnight.

**3.** Remove astragalus, add water to bring back up to 4 cups, add rice, and bring to a boil.

**4.** Reduce heat and simmer until done, approximately 1 hour.

---

## BONESET *(Eupatorium perfoliatum)*

**Family:** Compositae.

**Part used:** Above-ground plant.

**Collection and habitat:** Indigenous to North America. If allowed to dry, the flowering plant will usually go to seed. The plant should be collected while in flower (August or September) if tincture is to be made from fresh herb. Otherwise, it should be picked just before flowering, hung upside down in a shaded place, and allowed to air-dry thoroughly.

**Actions:** Immunostimulant (increases phagocytosis to 4 times that seen with echinacea), diaphoretic, febrifuge, mucous membrane tonic, smooth-muscle relaxant, anti-inflammatory, cytotoxic, mild emetic, peripheral circulatory stimulant, gastric bitter.

**Function in liver disease:** Boneset has been used for centuries to treat dengue fever caused by a virus that is closely related to HCV. Boneset is good at alleviating the intermittent fevers and chills that are common with HCV infection. Boneset is strongly analgesic and is exceptionally stimulating to the immune system.

## About Boneset

The plant was extensively used by native peoples for hundreds if not thousands of years, specifically for intermittent fevers and chills accompanied by pain in the bones, weakness, and debility.

Clinical trials have shown that boneset stimulates phagocytosis better than echinacea, is analgesic (it is at least as effective as aspirin), and alleviates cold and flu symptoms. In mice, it has shown strong immunostimulant activity and cytotoxic action against cancer cells.

Despite boneset's long history of use, the herb has not fully come back into vogue. Little research has been done on it, especially with regard to treatment of liver disease. Nonetheless, boneset has long been used for chronic liver problems, in part because chronic liver disease often results in impaired immune functioning and intermittent fever and chills. Matthew Wood comments that "boneset is most commonly used for debility from old intermittants [diseases causing fever and chills] which have damaged the tension on the gallbladder reflexes and caused problems due to wrongs of the bilious apparatus. . . . It is an admirable tonic to restore the appetite especially in alcoholics whose appetite has been ruined by drinking."

I have found it one of the best of the "undiscovered" herbal medicines and believe it is of especial benefit for hepatitis and chronic liver disease. Echinacea tincture (30–60 drops up to 6 times per day for acute conditions) may be used as an alternative.

## Preparation and Dosage

May be taken as a tea or tincture.

**Tea:** *Cold* — 1 ounce (30 mL) herb in quart (L) boiling water, let steep overnight. Strain and drink throughout day. The cold infusion is better for the mucous membrane system and as a liver tonic. *Hot* — 1 tsp (5 mL) herb in 8 ounces (240 mL) hot water, steep 15 minutes. Take 4–6 ounces (120–180 mL) up to 4 times per day.

**Note:** Boneset is only a diaphoretic when hot, and it should be consumed hot for active infections or for recurring chills and fevers.

**Tincture:** *Fresh herb in flower:* 1:2 in 95 percent alcohol, 20–40 drops up to 3 times per day in hot water. *Dry herb:* 1:5 in 60 percent alcohol, 30–50 drops in hot water up to 3 times per day. *For acute viral or bacterial upper respiratory tract infections:* 10 drops of tincture in hot water every half-hour up to 6 times per day. For chronic conditions in which the acute stage has passed but chronic fatigue and relapse continue: 10 drops of tincture in 8 ounces (240 mL) hot water 4 times per day.

## Contraindications and Side Effects

Hot infusion in large quantities can cause vomiting; otherwise, there are no side effects. It has been erroneously reported that the fresh plant contains trematol, which causes "milk sickness" in cows and people who drink infected milk. My research shows that trematol is confined to *Eupatorium rugosum* and white snakeroot and does not occur in boneset. Many clinicians feel that tincture is best made with fresh boneset and that the dried herb should be used for tea.

# CODONOPSIS *(Codonopsis pilosula,* et al.)

**Family:** Campanulaceae.

**Part used:** Root.

**Collection and habitat:** There are over 40 species of codonopsis, about 20 of which have been used as "codonopsis" in herbal medicine, primarily in China. Several species of codonopsis are grown as rock garden ornamentals in the United States and Europe.

Roots older than 3 years are harvested in September or October. The roots are half-dried in the sun and then rubbed by hand on a board until the root tissue compresses. They are then dried two-thirds of the way and rubbed again. At that point, they are dried completely in the sun. Foster suggests breaking the roots open and checking the interior for black color. If the interior is not black, the root is well prepared.

**Actions:** Immune and spleen tonic and potentiator, antioxidant, anti-inflammatory, cardiotonic, antiulcer, astringent, analgesic, antidyspeptic.

**Functions in liver disease:** Alleviates fatigue, weakness, dizziness, facial swelling, and lack of appetite; acts as immune tonic; increases endurance; serves as an antistressor and antihepatotoxic.

## About Codonopsis

Codonopsis first became known in the 18th century in China, where it quickly took its place as "the poor man's ginseng." It is considered specific for fatigue, weakness, loss of appetite, vertigo, dyspepsia, nephritis, and spleen insufficiency in Chinese medicine.

Codonopsis has shown stronger antioxidant activity than *Panax ginseng* in vitro, as well as strong anti-inflammatory and antispasmodic action. In vivo studies have reported strong analgesic, anti-inflammatory, antiulcer, and hypotensive action. Codonopsis has shown consistent hepatoprotective activity against $CCl_4$-induced hepatotoxicity in vivo, as well as antitumor activity. The herb was also found to have strong immunostimulant activity in protecting guinea pigs from cobra venom: It increased complement and neutrophil phagocytosis. Laboratory studies indicate that codonopsis enhances phagocytosis of the reticuloendothelial system (especially that of the Kupffer cells in the liver), thus enhancing and strengthening the immune system and the liver's ability to process toxins from the blood.

Codonopsis has been effectively used in combination formulas in clinical trials for chronic bronchitis, myocardial infarction, cataracts, AIDS, uterine hemorrhage, heart failure, and scleroderma.

## Preparation and Dosage

Used as a powder or in capsules.

**Powder:** The powder may be made into a tea or strong decoction and consumed daily if desired. The root is often ground into flour and used in cooking in China.

**Capsules:** 6–15 g (12–30 "00" capsules) when used in combination with other herbs, 30–60 g (1–2 ounces) per day when used alone.

## Contraindications and Side Effects

None noted.

## LICORICE  *(Glycyrrhiza glabra)*

**Family:** Leguminosae.
**Part used:** Root.
**Collection and habitat:** *Glycyrrhiza glabra* is a native of Europe and is usually commercially grown and hence purchased from retail or whole-sale suppliers. It does not grow wild in North America, although another related species is widely found here (it is not very sweet but can be used in like fashion). Usually picked in early spring or fall when the leaves begin to die back. Because of the high levels of environmental pollution in eastern Europe, where most commercial licorice is grown, only organic licorice should be purchased for use.
**Actions:** Antioxidant, antidiuretic, smooth-muscle relaxant, antispas-modic, immunostimulant (stimulates interferon production; enhances antibody formation; stimulates phagocytosis; acts as antistressor, adrenal tonic, thymus stimulant), antiulcer, anti-inflammatory, tumor inhibitor, free-radical inhibitor, antihepatotoxic, antimalarial, gentle laxative, expectorant, demulcent, anticardiotoxic, immunomodulator, analgesic, antihyperglycemic. Also protects from effects of radiation exposure, reduces gastric secretions, and stimulates pancreatic secretions.
**Functions in liver disease:** Antistressor, immune system stimulant, adrenal tonic, thymus tonic; hepatoprotective, anti-inflammatory, antiviral.

## About Licorice

Licorice is a remarkable herb. Generally, it is an immune system stimu-lant that has impressive antibacterial, antiviral, antitumor, and antiulcer activity and potentiates the actions of other herbs. One distinct advan-tage of licorice is its sweetness. Licorice is 50 times sweeter than sugar and, when used in herbal combinations, helps brighten the awful taste accompanying many herbal formulations.

Licorice has a long history of clinical human trials; its side effects and strengths are well documented. It is specific for upper respiratory tract infections, coughs, colds, and ulcerations anywhere in the gastrointestinal tract, especially the stomach. Scientific studies have shown that it increases the generation and aggressiveness of white blood cells, stimulates interferon production in the body, and enhances antibody formation. Several trials have reported that it also possesses distinct immunomodulator activity: If the immune system is overactive, licorice calms it down; if the immune system is underactive, licorice pumps it up.

A related species, *G. uralensis,* has shown antiviral activity against HBV in vitro. This species has also been found to have broad liver-protective actions against hepatotoxicity induced by ethanol and $CCl_4$. In vivo, *G. glabra* lowers liver enzyme levels that have been elevated by cholic acid and poor diet. One active constituent of all licorice species is glycyrrhizin. A recent study in Japan found that glycyrrhizin inhibited the development of liver cancer from hepatitis. Steven Foster comments that "licorice has been used in modern China for the treatment of chronic viral hepatitis with over a 70 percent success rate. Preparations are given over a period of two or three months, resulting in improvement of symptoms such as malaise, anorexia, abdominal distention, nausea, and vomiting. Improvement of liver function tests and a reduction in the size of an enlarged liver or spleen has been observed." The Japanese have patented an injectable licorice extract that is used by prescription for treatment of HCV infection.

Licorice has shown distinct antifatigue and antistress activity, and in vivo studies have reported strong activity against cancerous tumors and a protective effect from the effects of radiation. Perhaps licorice is best known for two things: its estrogenic effects, which make it a useful herb for menopause, and its antiulcer activity, which makes it an herb of choice for both stomach and duodenal ulceration. Because it stimulates expectoration and is powerfully healing for mucous membrane systems, it has a long history of use for upper respiratory tract infections.

## Preparation and Dosage

Used as tincture, tea, capsule, and powder.

**Tincture:** Dried root, 1:5 in 50 percent alcohol, 30–60 drops up to 3 times per day.

**Tea:** ½–1 tsp (2.5–5 mL) powdered root in 8 ounces (240 mL) water, simmer 15 minutes, strain. Up to 3 cups per day.

**Capsules:** 2–8 "00" capsules per day.

**Powder:** 1–2 tsp (10 mL) per day.

### Contraindications and Side Effects

Many. Because of licorice's many strengths, people sometimes overuse it, occasionally with serious side effects. Overdoses or long use of high doses can cause severe potassium depletion (hypokalemia); hypertension; decrease in plasma renin and aldosterone levels; edema; and, at very high doses, decreased body and thymus weight and reduced blood cell counts. Because of licorice's strong estrogenic activity, it also causes breast growth in men, especially when combined with other estrogenic herbs such as hops or black cohosh. Luckily, all these conditions tend to abate within 2 to 4 weeks after licorice intake ceases. The side effects seem to be limited to extracts; the whole root apparently is free of them. Still, caution should be used in choosing the length and strength of dosages.

Licorice is contraindicated in hypertension, hypokalemia, pregnancy, hypernatremia, and steroid use.

## PANAX (OR ASIAN) GINSENG (*Panax ginseng*)

**Family:** Araliaceae.

**Part used:** Generally, the root. The leaves, although milder in action, can also be used.

**Collection and habitat:** A native of eastern Asia (Korea, Russia, China), panax ginseng is rare in the wild because of overharvesting. Occasionally, plants over 100 years old are still found; these sell for up to $20,000 per ounce. The herb is now extensively commercially cultivated; the roots are harvested in the fall of the fifth year. The older the roots, the better medicines they are considered to be.

**Actions:** Tonic, adaptogen, stimulant, immunomodulator, immune system stimulant, blood pressure and sugar regulator, cerebral circulation stimulant, cognitive function enhancer, adrenal tonic, antitumor.

**Functions in liver disease:** Helps alleviate general weakness, fatigue, low libido, exhaustion, brain fog, and lack of appetite. Enhances immune function, interferon production, and phagocytosis. Modulates white blood cell counts. Potentiates almost all liver functions, including RNA and DNA repair and production of vital proteins. Lowers liver enzyme levels in the blood. Hepatoprotective, antiviral, antitumor.

## About Panax Ginseng

Panax ginseng is probably the most famous of Chinese herbs and has been used in TCM for thousands of years. It has been administered alone or in combination for general weakness, sexual debility, lack of appetite, anemia, forgetfulness, immune deficiency, high and low blood pressure, and adrenal deficiency. Medical research on ginseng can and does fill several large volumes with exceptionally tiny type. What follows is only a sample of the problems associated with hepatitis. In both human and laboratory studies, ginseng has been found to be strongly protective of the liver, to lower liver enzyme levels, to positively affect cholesterol and lipid metabolism, and to be radioprotective, antitumor, antioxidant, and antiviral.

Panax ginseng has shown antiviral activity in vitro against HBV. One human trial reported that ginseng, along with multivitamins, can significantly reduce chronic liver disease in elderly patients within 12 weeks. Ginseng has been shown to be hepatoprotective in vivo against liver disease induced by $CCl_4$, chloroform, galactosamine, and ethanol. Other in vivo studies showed that it protected the liver from ethanol-induced hyperlipidemia. It also reduced cellular swelling, congestion, bile pigmentation, and elevated aminotransferase levels; reduced liver enzyme levels; prevented dexamethasone-induced increases in amino-transferase levels; and protected against ethanol-induced mitochondrial swelling and disruption, pyknosis and fat deposition, depression of phospholipid synthesis, and stimulation of triglyceride synthesis. A combination of ginseng and bupleurum given in vivo before $CCl_4$ injection significantly reduced cellular-level liver damage in mice.

More than 500 published scientific papers have addressed the actions of ginseng. Some of the most noted areas of activity concern the herb's immune-enhancing, radioprotective, and antitumor properties.

Ginseng has been found to enhance antibody response, natural killer cell action, interferon production, and overall power and strength of the immune system. Many studies on the use of ginseng in cancer treatment in China showed that ginseng possesses strong antitumor actions. Treated panax (called red or kirin ginseng) showed the strongest activity. Ginseng has also been reported to have a strong ability to protect living organisms from the effects of radiation.

### Preparation and Dosage

As powder or tincture.
**Powder:** 1–2 tsp (5–10 mL) per day.
**Tincture:** 1:5 in 70 percent alcohol. White root, 20–40 drops; red cured root (Chinese of Korean), 5–20 drops, both up to 3 times per day. American species *(Panax quinquefolium)*: woodsgrown, 10–20 drops up to 3 times per day.

### Contraindications and Side Effects

Men younger than age 40 should use Siberian ginseng, not panax ginseng. Contraindicated in high blood pressure, excessive menstrual bleeding, and pregnancy. May cause high blood pressure, irritability, insomnia, muscle tension, headache, and restlessness.

## RED ROOT (*Ceanothus* spp.)

**Family:** Rhamnaceae.
**Part used:** The root or inner bark of the root. The various species of red root can be used interchangeably.
**Collection and habitat:** Species seem to grow everywhere and are widely divergent in appearance. The root should be harvested in the fall or early spring, whenever the root has been subjected to a good frost. The inner bark of the root is bright red, and this color extends through the white woody root as a pink tinge after a freeze. The root is extremely tough when it dries. It should be cut into small 1- or 2-inch (2.5 or 5 cm) pieces with plant snips while still fresh.

**Actions:** First and foremost, a lymph system stimulant and tonic. Anti-inflammatory for liver and spleen. It is also an astringent, a mucous membrane tonic, and an exceptionally strong blood coagulant; alterative, antiseptic, expectorant, antispasmodic.

**Functions in liver disease:** Reducing inflammation in liver and spleen, stimulating lymph system clearance and drainage, helping clear hepatitis viruses from lymph system.

## About Red Root

Red root is an important herb because it helps facilitate clearing of dead cellular tissue from the lymph system. When the immune system is responding to acute conditions or the onset of disease, as white blood cells kill disease pathogens they are taken to the lymph system for disposal. When the lymph system can clear out dead cellular material rapidly, the healing process is increased, sometimes dramatically. The herb shows especially strong action whenever any portion of the lymph system is swollen, infected, or inflamed. This includes the lymph nodes, tonsils (entire back of throat), spleen, appendix, and liver. Some evidence suggests that red root's activity in the lymph nodes also enhances the lymph nodes' production of lymphocytes, specifically the formation of T cells. Clinicians working with AIDS patients, who historically have low T-cell counts, have noted increases after the use of red root. Nineteenth-century western botanic medicine used the herb to reduce inflammations in the liver and spleen.

A number of human trials have used the herb as a tincture extract (usually ⅓–½ oz [10–15 mL] per person). The trials focused on heavy bleeding, including excess menstruation, and found that red root was a powerful coagulant and hemostatic. Clotting time was also reduced. In vivo studies have shown marked hemostatic activity and hypotensive action. In vitro studies have reported a strong reverse transcriptase inhibition and broad antifungal activity.

## Preparation and Dosage

As tincture, tea, strong decoction, or gargle or in capsules.

**Tincture:** Dried root, 1:5 in 50 percent alcohol, 30–90 drops up to 4 times per day.

**Tea:** 1 tsp (5 mL) powdered root in 8 ounces (240 mL) water, simmer 15 minutes, strain. Up to 6 cups per day.

**Strong decoction:** 1 ounce (30 mL) herb in 16 ounces (480 mL) water, cover, and simmer slowly 30 minutes. One tbs (15 mL) 3 or 4 times per day.

**Gargle:** For tonsillitis or throat inflammations, gargle with strong tea 4–6 times per day.

**Capsules:** 10–30 "00" capsules per day.

### Contraindications and Side Effects

No side effects noted, but red root is contraindicated in people using blood coagulants or anticoagulants and in pregnant women.

## SCHIZANDRA *(Schisandra chinensis)*

**Family:** Schisandraceae

**Part used:** Usually the fruit, although sometimes the whole plant is used.

**Collection and habitat:** The plant, a woody aromatic vine, is native to Manchuria, China, and Japan. Generally, the berries are considered the primary medicine and are harvested when ripe in late summer or early fall. They are usually dried and are traditionally used as decoctions or infusions.

**Actions:** General tonic, immune restorative, adaptogenic, rejuvenative, antioxidant, antihepatotoxic, hepatoprotective, detoxifier, antitussive, demulcent, antioxidant, sexual tonic.

**Functions in liver disease:** Antihepatotoxic; liver detoxifier; increases nonspecific resistance; reduces liver enzyme levels (specifically alanine aminotransferase); increases liver protein and glycogen synthesis; helps prevent liver cancer; enhances glutathione production; helps reverse fatigue, insomnia, weakness, depression, and forgetfulness.

### About Schizandra

For at least 2000 years, schizandra has been used in Chinese medicine, where it is called "wu wei dze." Schizandra has a lengthy history of use in Asia as a restorative for the immune system, a liver tonic, an adaptogenic, and a treatment for fatigue, weakness, depression, forgetfulness, and insomnia. It is also considered a good astringent and promotes semen production. Modern research and contemporary clinical use have borne out its immune-potentiating and adaptogenic actions, in addition to revealing its strong actions as a liver protectant and treatment for hepatitis C.

One clinical trial in China of 189 cases of chronic hepatitis C found that in patients who received schizandra fruit, alanine aminotransferase levels returned to normal faster than in controls. Liver protein and glycogen synthesis were increased. Another human study found that nonspecific resistance was increased. Steven Foster comments that "alcohol extracts have helped to regenerate liver tissue, and thus have been used clinically for hepatitis. Chinese researchers have isolated a number of lignins from the fruits of Schisandra. At least 13 lignin compounds from five species of schisandra have shown the ability to lower elevated levels of . . . SGPT [alanine aminotransferase]. . . . The drug has been tested in over 5,000 cases of hepatitis patients with success rates from 84 to 97.9 percent in lowering SGPT levels." He reports that for nonjaundiced infectious hepatitis, the dried baked powder of the fruits is used in 3 g doses 3 times per day until alanine aminotransferase levels return to normal; use then continues for another 2 to 4 weeks. If symptoms return after treatment is discontinued, the dosage is raised. In one trial of 102 patients, after 30 days of treatment 76 percent of patients reported significant improvement and 85.3 percent reported some improvement.

In vivo studies have shown that schizandra stimulates glutathione-S-transferase induction; prevents DNA binding of aflatoxin B1; and is antihepatotoxic, protecting the liver from $CCl_4$, chloroform, acetaminophen, galactosamine, gossypol acetic acid, and thioacetamide and lowering both alanine aminotransferase and aspartate aminotransferase levels. Numerous other studies have reported consistent alanine aminotransferase–lowering action upon administration of schizandra and consistent inhibition of any increase in aspartate aminotransferase levels upon administration of liver toxins.

In vivo, schizandra prevents glutathione depletion; stimulates glutathione production; stimulates glycogenesis; inhibits lipid peroxide formation; stimulates the cytochrome P450 enzyme system; is strongly active against liver flukes; inhibits aspartate aminotransferase; inhibits glutamate-oxaloacetate-aminotransferase; inhibits creatinine phosphokinase; stimulates glucose-6-phosphate dehydrogenase; enhances memory; stimulates nonspecific resistance; is an immunomodulator; and is adaptogenic.

In vitro research has shown a strong superoxide radical–scavenging effect (tincture of decoction residue) and antioxidant and antihepatotoxic action against numerous liver toxins.

## Preparation and Dosage

May be taken as infusion or decoction, powder or capsules, or tincture.
**Infusion or decoction**: 2–6 g in 8 ounces (240 mL) water per day.
**Loose powder or capsules**: 2–6 g (4–12 "00" capsules) per day.
**Tincture:** 1:5 in 70 percent alcohol up to 1 tsp (5 mL) 3 times per day.

## Contraindications and Side Effects

None.

## SIBERIAN GINSENG *(Eleutherococcus senticosus)*

**Family:** Araliaceae.
**Part used:** Root.
**Collection and habitat:** The plant is indigenous to northeast Asia but is now being grown commercially in a few places in the United States. It is usually purchased commercially, with the root already cut and sifted to industry standards.
**Actions:** Adaptogen, antistressor, immune tonic, immunopotentiating, immunoadjuvant; increases nonspecific resistance against many pathogens; monoamine oxidase inhibitor.
**Functions in liver disease:** Antistressor, immune tonic and potentiator (stimulates B lymphocyte antibodies), antidepressant, mental clarity stimulant; helps restore task endurance.

## About Siberian Ginseng

Although used in China for several thousand years, this herb was brought to prominence by intensive Russian research in the latter half of the 20th century. Many clinical trials have shown significant immune-enhancing activity. This includes significant increase in immunocompetent cells, specifically T lymphocytes (helper/inducers, cytotoxic, and natural killer cells). Tests of the herb have repeatedly shown that it increases the ability of humans to withstand adverse conditions, increases mental alertness, and improves performance. People taking the herb regularly report fewer illnesses than people not taking it.

In general, Siberian ginseng is completely nontoxic, and Russian investigators have reported on use of exceptionally large doses for up to 20 years with no adverse reactions. Both Asian and American ginseng, on the other hand, have several limitations. Siberian ginseng, in my experience, produces cumulative results: The longer you use it, the better it works. It tends to kick in after 6 weeks or so, and the most significant results can be seen after 6 months of use. This is especially true in people with pale, unhealthy skin; lassitude; and depression.

*Eleutherococcus senticosus* and a related species, *E. chiisanensis,* have been found to be strongly antihepatotoxic and hepatoprotective in vivo against $CCl_4$-induced hepatotoxicity. Additionally, Siberian ginseng was found to be a hepatoregenerator, significantly stimulating liver regeneration in animals in which portions of the liver had been surgically removed.

Because Siberian ginseng is a monoamine oxidase inhibitor, it is also useful for depression, a condition that often accompanies a severely depleted immune system and chronic liver disease.

### Preparation and Dosage

Used as tea, tincture, or powder or in capsules.

**Tea:** Cold infusion, 3–6 ounces (90–180 mL) up to 3 times per day

**Tincture:** Dried herb: 1:5 in 60 percent alcohol, 20–60 drops up to 3 times per day.

**Powder:** 1–2 tsp (5–10 mL) per day.

**Capsules:** 2 "00" capsules 3 times per day.

*Note:* The Russian studies were carried out on a 1:1 extract in 30 percent alcohol, 2–15 ml in a daily dose. This is a much stronger dose than that described above and works more quickly. Numerous herbal companies produce it in this form.

## Contraindications and Side Effects

For almost all people, there are no side effects or contraindications. The herb may temporarily increase blood pressure in some people. This increased pressure tends to drop to normal within a few weeks. Caution should be exercised for people with very high blood pressure, especially if the herb is combined with other hypertensives, such as licorice. With extreme overuse, tension and insomnia may occur.

## TIENCHI GINSENG *(Panax pseudoginseng,* var. *notoginseng,* var. *japonicus)*

**Family:** Araliaceae.
**Part used:** Root.
**Collection and habitat:** An Asian herb used primarily in Korea, China, and Japan; the root is gathered in the spring or fall. The older the roots, the better.
**Actions:** Immune tonic and stimulant, adaptogenic, hepatoprotective, antiviral, cardiotonic, anti-inflammatory, anticomplement, antihyperglycemic, antiulcer, antioxidant, hemostatic, analgesic; promotes blood circulation.
**Functions in liver disease:** Antiviral, hepatoprotective, strong stimulant and tonic for the immune system. Directly active against hepatitis viruses.

## About Tienchi Ginseng

In the literature, two species are considered to be *Panax pseudoginseng:* 1) *Panax notoginseng* or *P. pseudoginseng* var. *notoginseng* ("san qi") and 2) *P. japonicus* or *P. pseudoginseng* var. *japonicus* (and even more confusing, two subspecies: *P. japonicus* var. *major* or var. *bipinnatifidus*), which is also called "zhu-jie-shen." The species have been found to have nearly identical actions in scientific studies, although their traditional uses vary. Some practitioners consider them both to be "tienchi" ginseng, whereas others assert that only *P. notoginseng* should be called "tienchi." Research for both is included here under the name "tienchi."

Tienchi ginseng is considered specific for the liver and stomach in Chinese medicine. Extensive research has been conducted on tienchi, and some strong responses have been reported in the treatment of hepatitis and immune functioning.

One clinical trial used an 80 percent alcohol extract administered intravenously (1.2 g per person per day) to 40 patients with hepatitis who had had elevated alanine aminotransferase levels for 6 months and had not responded to other treatments. Daily dosing was given for up to 6 months depending on the patient; 31 of 40 patients eventually had normal liver function test results and no signs of hepatitis. Several other clinical studies used multicomponent herbal mixtures as hot decoctions (10.4 g per day) and found that triglyceride, cholesterol, and LDL levels decreased dramatically, whereas HDL levels rose. (The mix was composed of *Polygonum multiflorum, Polygonum cuspidatum, Alisma plantago-aquatica, Rheum tanguticum,* and *Panax pseudoginseng*). External application in clinical studies has shown a significant antipruritic action (anti-itching) and hair-stimulant effect. Of interest, one of the primary actions of strongly protective and regenerative liver herbs seems to be hair-growth or hair-stimulant action; one of the side effects of severe liver disease can be hair loss.

In vitro studies in China and Japan have shown that tienchi has direct antiviral activity against HBV. Tienchi has also been found in vitro to inhibit the Epstein-Barr virus.

In vivo studies have reported antihepatotoxic activity against liver damage induced by $CCl_4$, galactosamine, and lipopolysaccharide; choleretic action; inhibition of lipid peroxide formation; and stimulation of superoxide dismutase. Tienchi inhibits glutamate pyruvate aminotransferase; stimulates protein synthesis (incorporation of (3H)-thymidine into liver DNA and (3H)-leucine into both the liver and serum proteins was significantly improved in $CCl_4$-treated animals); has strong antihypercholesterolemic and antihypertriglyceridemic action; alleviates brain edemas; is strongly anti-inflammatory; and is strongly cytotoxic and antitumor. Some of its strongest activity has been shown in vivo with regard to its effects on the heart and blood. It is strongly cardiotonic (preventing induced arrhythmias and myocardial damage) and enhances blood flow to and from the heart and brain. It has also been shown to be adaptogenic and an immunostimulant, with a pronounced radical scavenging effect; to inhibit platelet aggregation; and to stimulate gamma-interferon production. It was also found to consistently inhibit ulcers and to provide strong analgesic action.

## Preparation and Dosage

As capsules, tincture, or tea.
**Capsules:** 1–15 "00" capsules per day.
**Tincture:** 1:5 in 70 percent alcohol, 25–75 drops per day (1–3 mL).
**In Chinese medicine,** 1–2 g powder is used; for infusion or decoction (tea), 5–10 g is used.

## Contraindications and Side Effects

None.

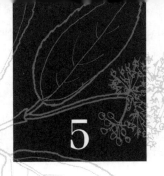

# NUTRITIONAL SUPPLEMENTS FOR HEPATITIS C

Many nutritional supplements have been found to be extremely helpful in treating viral hepatitis. These supplements stimulate and support the immune system, enhance energy levels, facilitate faster healing time, support liver health, and reverse liver damage. Evidence also strongly suggests that several of these supplements protect the body against liver cirrhosis and cancer and provide actual antiviral activity against HCV.

## ALPHA-LIPOIC ACID (ALA)

**Actions:** Antioxidant, chelation agent, radioprotective, enzymatic catalyst, glutathione production stimulant, neurotonic, antiviral; normalizes blood sugar levels.

**Functions in liver disease:** Immunostimulant, liver protector, liver regenerator, enhances memory and mental clarity, reduces inflammation in joints, enhances energy levels, reduces risk of liver cancer.

**About ALA:** ALA was isolated in 1951 from liver tissue. It turns out that human cells, especially in the liver, naturally produce ALA, although as we grow older we make less and less of it. ALA is vitally important in numerous bodily systems. Its two most important characteristics are its intracellular antioxidant and detoxification activity and its ability to stimulate the production of glutathione, a vital substance in preventing viral replication and an essential detoxification substance in its own right. ALA is so small that it acts to detoxify cells both from within and without. (Vitamin C is so large that it can act only on the outside of cells.) ALA actually helps protect our cells from damage at the genetic level.

> ## Top Seven Nutritional Supplements for Hepatitis C
>
> Alpha-lipoic acid
> *N*-acetylcysteine
> Selenium
> Vitamin B complex
> Vitamin C
> Vitamin E
> Zinc

ALA has shown remarkable liver-protective and -regenerative properties. Other than milk thistle and picrorhiza, ALA is the one substance found to protect the liver from the powerful toxins produced by *Amanita phalloides* mushrooms and even to stimulate regeneration of the liver itself. Burt Berkson, a physician in New Mexico, found that in severe cases of mushroom poisoning, liver enzyme levels returned to normal in as little as 2 weeks after ALA use. (Similar results have been obtained in studies in Sweden and elsewhere.) Berkson reported that when ALA was used with milk thistle, liver damage from hepatitis C was reversed and liver enzyme levels returned to normal.

German researchers have found ALA to be effective in treatment of AIDS patients. After 14 days, plasma ascorbate and glutathione levels increased, markers of plasma lipid peroxidation decreased, and T-helper cells increased in half the patients. In vitro studies have shown activity of ALA against several viruses, including HIV. ALA has been reported to reduce viral load in people infected with HIV.

Studies of people exposed to radiation indicate that ALA protects the liver, brain, skin, and heart against lipid peroxidation. The most dramatic protection occurs in the liver.

In several studies, ALA enhanced memory, presumably by improving *N*-methyl-o-aspartate receptor density (it produced no effects in young laboratory animals). This capacity for enhancing mental clarity and memory has also been seen in humans.

ALA has shown remarkable effects in helping diabetic patients by normalizing blood sugar levels. It increases glucose uptake by muscle cells, leading to more energy, and stimulates muscle recovery and tone. It has also shown a marked ability to protect the neural network of the body from disease, to ease nerve pain, and, in some cases, to restore damaged nerves.

**Dosage:** *Maintenance dosage:* 50–100 mg per day. *For acute or chronic disease:* 300 mg 2 times per day; 600 mg doses in many instances showed better results than 1000 or 1200 mg doses. ALA is available at most health food stores and pharmacies.

**Contraindications and Side Effects:** None noted at normal doses. High levels of ALA can cause some side effects, especially at doses over 1800 mg per day. However, the toxic dose is over 30 g, making the recommended dosages very safe for internal use. Diabetic patients should use ALA only after review with their physician because ALA strongly affects blood sugar levels and will throw off any medical protocols that are in place.

## N-Acetylcysteine (NAC)

**Actions:** Antioxidant, hepatoprotective, immunomodulator, antiviral, anticarcinogenic; increases glutathione levels.

**Functions in liver disease:** Immunostimulant, liver protector, possibly antiviral against HCV; normalizes immune functioning, inhibits formation of liver cancer, is synergistic with interferon.

**About NAC:** NAC is a glutathione precursor. As it is metabolized in the body, it is converted into glutathione. Research suggests that glutathione is most effective if it is made by the body, not taken as a supplement. Because of this, NAC is crucial in the diet, especially for those with depletion levels. Glutathione itself is strongly liver protective, activates killer lymphocytes, potentiates interferon activity in the body, and represses viral replication. The U.S. poison control centers recommend NAC as the primary treatment to protect the liver from Tylenol (acetaminophen) poisoning.

Researchers in Spain found that in 41 percent of patients with HCV infection who had not responded to interferon therapy and were re-treated with the addition of NAC, alanine aminotransferase levels decreased to normal. Levels in the remaining patients significantly declined.

Several studies have reported that patients with HIV infection and those with HCV infection have significantly lower levels of glutathione. In AIDS patients, increases in glutathione levels induced by administration of NAC produced significant increases in survival times. In HIV-infected patients, 3000 mg of NAC given intravenously seemed to produce antiviral effects against HIV, significantly reducing viral loads. This finding supports results of in vitro studies that found NAC to be specifically active against HIV.

Other researchers have reported a definite and strong hepatoprotective effect from NAC. Eighty percent of rats that were given the powerful aflatoxin B1, which usually produces liver cancer, survived as long as 2 years with no detectable damage to their livers if they were first treated with NAC.

**Dosage:** 500–600 mg 3 times per day, taken with food. The action of NAC is enhanced by the presence of vitamin C, zinc, and selenium.

**Contraindications and Side Effects:** May aggravate stomach ulcers. If the liver is severely damaged, take glutathione instead. Diabetic patients should consult their physician before using NAC. Metabolism of NAC uses up minerals in the body, especially zinc and copper. Take with supplemental chelated zinc, copper added.

## ⊛Selenium

**Actions:** Antitumor, immune enhancer, antioxidant, detoxifier.

**Functions in liver disease:** Necessary for effective functioning of glutathione peroxidase, which helps detoxify the body, protects cellular DNA from carcinogens (helping prevent liver cancer), and stimulates immune and thyroid function.

**About Selenium:** Perhaps the most important recent discovery about HCV is that it (and a number of other viruses, such as HIV, EBV, and HHV6) destroys (or lyses) selenium. As the disease develops, selenium levels in the body fall. As levels fall the body begins to use more and more glutathione and vitamin E (with which selenium often combines), leading to depletions in both those important nutrients. Selenium deficiency itself can cause liver cirrhosis. Because HCV destroys such large amounts of selenium, it is important to add selenium as a supplement to the diet.

**Dosage:** 50–200 mcg per day. During active liver disease the suggested dosage is 200 mcg per day.

**Contraindications and side effects:** Selenium can be extremely toxic causing nausea, vomiting, liver and heart damage at high levels. It is important to not exceed 200 mcg per day.

# VITAMIN B COMPLEX

**Actions:** The complex of B vitamins are hepatoprotective and anti-inflammatory, improve hepatic function, stimulate the immune system, act as a tonic to the spleen and liver, and aid fat metabolism.

**Functions in liver disease:** The B vitamin complex supports the cytochrome P450 system, which regulates the liver's detoxification processes, enhances spleen function, reduces arthritis inflammation, decreases fatigue, supports healthy adrenal function, helps improve appetite, enhances energy levels and mental clarity, supports T-cell function, controls eczema, and helps fat metabolism.

**About Vitamin B Complex:** Vitamin B complex is often deficient in people with HCV. Since low levels of vitamin B result in many of the symptoms reported by people with HCV infection, it makes sense to take a good supplement daily. Taking a supplement is especially important for helping the liver perform its detoxification processes.

**Dosage:** Take 1–2 tablets of a standard B complex formulation per day. Follow directions on bottle.

**Contraindications and Side Effects:** Excess vitamin B complex is excreted in the urine and will turn urine bright yellow. Because your body needs more vitamin B complex from time to time, urine will become paler and then brighten again. Extremely high doses may cause headache.

# VITAMIN C

**Actions:** Antioxidant, immune system potentiator, wound healing accelerator, collagen production enhancer.

**Functions in liver disease:** Speeds up healing time, strengthens immune system, enhances action of NAC, protects tissue from effects of free radicals, may be antiviral and anticarcinogenic.

**About Vitamin C:** Most animals, with the exception of humans and other primates, make their own vitamin C. As is now well known, vitamin C is essential to prevent scurvy and other deficiency diseases. However, it also speeds up healing time in most diseases and surgeries, enhances immune function, and protects the body from the effects of free radicals.

Some evidence suggests that vitamin C is antiviral at large doses, although this has not been tested in cases of HCV infection. Long-standing evidence indicates that in some instances it helps prevent or even cure some cancers.

Robert Myers, a naturopathic physician in Arizona, has been using intravenous vitamin C in patients with viral hepatitis (HAV, HBV, and HCV), with excellent results. He uses 30 to 50 g, 1 g of calcium, 1 g of magnesium, and 2000 micrograms of vitamin $B_{12}$ in an intravenous drip given 3 times per week for 1 week. The whole regime is then repeated 30 days later. Myers reports that normal energy levels returned and liver enzyme levels normalized, on average, within 1 to 2 weeks. Responses in patients with hepatitis of long duration or hepatitis caused by aggressive viral subtypes take longer.

**Dosage:** Effervescent C-salts (the suggested form), ½ tsp (3–4 g) 2 times per day or to bowel tolerance. Vitamin C may also be taken in tablet form if desired.

**Contraindications and Side Effects:** Generally, vitamin C is prescribed "t.b.d." ("to bowel tolerance"). At higher levels, it causes flatulence and, eventually, diarrhea. Once you reach this level, back off slightly. This is the amount your body needs, which will fluctuate with your levels of health and stress. Vitamin C increases absorption of iron and is contraindicated at high doses for people with hemochromatosis (iron overload disease).

# Vitamin E

**Actions:** Antioxidant, immunopotentiator, anticirrhotic; synergistic with interferon; facilitates metabolism of fats.

**Functions in liver disease:** Protects the liver from oxidative stress, combats fatigue, boosts cell-mediated immunity, improves skin tone, prevents the molecular changes associated with cirrhosis, enhances interferon action in the body, reduces cholesterol levels in blood.

**About Vitamin E:** Lack of vitamin E causes cirrhosis, so the vitamin clearly plays a role in keeping liver cells healthy. Researchers at the University of California found that vitamin E actually prevents the molecular changes associated with cirrhosis. For anyone with chronic hepatitis C, in which there is a chance of cirrhosis, it makes sense to use this supplement. A study in Germany showed that 800 IU of vitamin E significantly improved liver enzyme levels in HCV-infected patients who were undergoing interferon therapy. Vitamin E also blocks oxidation of LDLs, preventing them from becoming harmful and raising cholesterol levels.

**Dosage:** *For persons under age 40:* 400 IU once per day; *for those over age 40:* 800 IU once per day. Take only natural vitamin E.

**Contraindications and Side Effects:** Take vitamin E with food to facilitate absorption; it may not be absorbed otherwise. No side effects have been noted, even at high doses.

# ZINC

**Actions:** Essential trace mineral for cell growth and replication; sexual maturity, fertility, and reproduction; healthy immune functioning; healthy skin and appetite; night vision.

**Functions in liver disease:** Promotes healthy thymus functioning (the "overseer" of the immune system), enhances strength and activity of natural killer cells (which specialize in attacking cancerous and virally infected cells), helps clear skin conditions often associated with liver disease, helps regulate blood sugar, assists in NAC metabolism, reverses the low zinc levels often accompanying liver disease.

**About Zinc:** Almost every cell of the body and hundreds of body enzymes contain zinc; it is stored in muscle and is concentrated in white and red blood cells, the prostate gland, nails, hair, eyes, liver, and skin. Low levels of zinc, common in liver disease, result in impaired thymus functioning (the thymus regulates the immune system as a whole), low activity of natural killer cells, decreased libido, poor skin health, and sleep disorders. Low levels of zinc also interfere with the body's ability to use glutathione efficiently.

**Dosage:** *General tonic dose for adults:* 20–25 mg per day. For acute or chronic conditions, 50 mg per day. A chelated brand is best, especially one with copper.

**Contraindications and Side Effects:** Very high doses can cause nausea, reduce HDL levels, raise cholesterol levels in the blood, cause skin rashes and depression, impair immunity, and create alcohol intolerance.

> ## Another Supplement
>
> Lactobrev, made from a fermented Japanese pickle, has been found to be one of the most effective stimulants of natural killer cells and interferon production in the body. The suggested dosage is 6–12 tablets per day 3 times per week. It may produce symptoms of flu (one of the symptoms of increased interferon production).

# CHANGING YOUR DIET:
# GIVING YOUR LIVER
# A BREAK

One of the most important things to do for treating hepatitis is reducing the work your liver has to do. One of the ways to do this is to eat foods that are easier for your liver to process, and to choose foods that are known to stimulate liver and immune health.

## RECOMMENDED FOODS

One of the best things you can do to reduce the stress on your liver is to alter your food intake for 10 weeks to allow your liver to rest and recuperate. Important elements of this diet change include low-fat foods, organic foods, and specific foods to help the liver heal.

Processing fats involves a lot of work for the liver, and in liver disease the liver may store unprocessed fats inside itself. Consuming a low-fat diet for 10 weeks alleviates a lot of the load and lets the liver rest and get better.

Organic food is imperative. The liver needs to work less, and residue from pesticides, fertilizers, antibiotics, and hormones makes it work very hard indeed.

Finally, many foods have been found to be exceptionally good for the liver.

> ### Four Major Foods for Hepatitis
>
> Bladderwrack
> Chlorella
> Green tea
> Spirulina

## WARNING ON PAIN MEDICATIONS

If you have hepatitis C, you should *never* take Tylenol or other forms of acetaminophen. Acetaminophen is exceptionally toxic to the liver and causes liver inflammation and failure. Unfortunately, this is the primary medication suggested by many physicians to alleviate the side effects of interferon therapy. All medications should be checked to see if they are contraindicated in the case of liver disease.

## BLADDERWRACK *(Fucus vesiculosus, F. distichus)*

**Family:** Fucaceae.
**Part used:** Whole plant.
**Collection and habitat:** Bladderwrack is a seaweed harvested throughout the year wherever it grows. It is usually dried and powdered for use, although it may be eaten whole as a sea vegetable.
**Actions:** Thyroid adaptogen, thyroid modulator, detoxification agent, antitumor agent, weight normalizer, nutrient (it is the major source of organic bioavailable iodine, trace elements, and minerals).
**Functions in liver disease:** Assisting in proper thyroid function and helping with weight normalization. Improves overall nutrition and lymphatic function. Helps remove or chelate toxic substances from the body. Buffers excess acidity in stomach and relieves nausea.

### About Bladderwrack

Bladderwrack is perhaps the primary food used to assist healthy functioning of the thyroid. The hormones produced by the thyroid regulate the metabolism in every cell of the body. When the body is under stress or extreme need, the thyroid, like the adrenal glands, produces and releases more hormones. However, under long-term stress or immune compromise the thyroid overloads and cannot keep up with demand. It begins to fail. Metabolism falls, depression sets in, much of the impetus for healthy liver functioning is lost, and the body temperature can begin to fall, leading to a constant feeling of chilliness. Other side effects are lethargy and decreased libido. Because of the importance of the thyroid in regulating cell metabolism, it is crucial that the thyroid in HCV-infected patients gets the important nutrients it needs.

Bladderwrack contains high concentrations of trace minerals, higher than in any land vegetable. It is a major source of iodine in a form that is easily usable by the body and contains D-iodotyrosine, a precursor needed for the thyroid's production of hormones. In the wild, bladderwrack is also symbiotic with a bacterium that produces minute quantities of thyroxine, a chemical synthesized by the thyroid gland that is often extracted and used to treat hypothyroidism (that is, a low-functioning thyroid gland).

**Preparation and Dosage:** Bladderwrack may be added to blended drinks (1–3 tsp [5–15 mL]), soups, or stews. It is often taken as a freeze-dried extract in capsules: 600 mg per day. The tincture tastes strongly of fish, and few people like it. As a tea, 2–3 tsp (10–15 mL) dried, powdered herb is used per cup of hot water. Let steep 10 minutes. One or more tsp (5 or more mL) of the powdered herb can be taken in juice each day.

**Contraindications and Side Effects:** Some people suggest that caution be used in patients with hyperthyroidism. However, in populations that eat bladderwrack in large quantities as a regular part of the diet, no problems associated with hyperthyroidism have been reported; the only exceptions are cases in which the bladderwrack was contaminated with industrial pollutants. Bladderwrack, like all sea vegetables, is as good as the water in which it is harvested. Buy only from sources that supply good-quality herbs.

Tablets are not suggested because the bladderwrack is subjected to high heat and other procedures in the manufacturing process. Many clinicians suggest using only nonprocessed bladderwrack or bladderwrack capsules.

## CHLORELLA *(Chlorella pyrendoidosa)*

**Family:** Chlorellaceae.

**Part used:** Chlorella is a one-celled green algae; the whole plant is used.

**Collection and habitat:** Chlorella grows in ponds and lakes and is generally commercially harvested. It has a strong cell wall that precludes human digestion; as a result, the cell wall is broken during processing so that chlorella can be used as a food.

**Actions:** Immunostimulant, nutrient, antitoxin, antitumor, cancer inhibitor, antioxidant; repairs DNA.

**Functions in liver disease:** Immunostimulant (increases interferon production and macrophage activity), nutrient (rich in chlorophyll, all essential amino acids, vitamins, and minerals), antiviral (active against HIV), antitumor; increases serum albumin levels.

## About Chlorella

Chlorella's great strengths lie in its abilities as a powerful nutrient substance, an immunostimulant, and an antitumor agent. Long-term in vivo, in vitro, and human studies have shown that chlorella stimulates macrophage activity, especially T and B cells. Through its activation of B cells, it stimulates the production of virus antibodies. One of the constituents of chlorella, chlorellan, stimulates interferon production in the body.

Chlorella is 58 percent protein and contains all the B vitamins, vitamins C and E, omega-3 fatty acids, and many minerals. Once the cell wall has been broken down, the nutrients in chlorella can be easily assimilated by the human body. The high protein content is especially good for people with liver disease. Chlorella stimulates growth and is beneficial for the severe weight loss that sometimes occurs with HCV infection. Several trials have shown chlorella's capacity to help people increase weight. This has been attributed to a constituent in chlorella called chlorella growth factor. Some of the factors in this substance have been found to help with depression, memory loss, and depleted energy levels, all problems associated with HCV infection. Because of the high levels of chlorophyll in chlorella, its use as a food stimulates the production of red blood cells. (Chemically, chlorophyll is nearly identical to hemoglobin.) Ingestion of supplemental chlorophyll has been found to be effective in speeding wound healing time. Chlorella also stimulates the production of white blood cells and serum albumin levels in the blood.

As an antitumor agent, chlorella is impressive. When directly injected into tumor sites or given as food, it has shown remarkable capacities to shrink existing tumors and significantly increase survival times. For persons at risk for liver cancer, it is an essential food to add to the diet.

**Preparation and Dosage:** *Take in tablet or powder form:* 1–5 tablets 3 times per day, 1–3 tbl (15–45 mL) powder per day.
**Contraindications and Side Effects:** No side effects noted, even with consumption of 1 pound (0.5 kg) per day as primary food source.

## GREEN TEA *(Camellia sinensis)*

**Family:** Theaceae.
**Part used:** Leaf.
**Collection and habitat:** Green tea is usually grown commercially in the Far East. After harvest, the fresh leaves are lightly steamed, then dried. Black tea is actually the fermented leaves of green tea.
**Actions:** Antitumor, cytotoxic; tumor inhibitor, hepatic detoxifier, antioxidant, immune system enhancer, hepatoprotector; enhances gap junction.
**Functions in liver disease:** Preventing or slowing liver cancer, protecting liver from toxin damage, stimulating immune system; beneficial in cholestasis through its ability to enhance gap junction; has antioxidant action and acts as a pick-me-up for combating fatigue.

### About Green Tea

Numerous studies have shown that green tea is an exceptionally strong antioxidant (four times stronger than black tea), inhibits cancer formation, lowers both cholesterol levels and blood pressure, is hepatoprotective, and is antibacterial and antiviral.

Green tea has been found in several in vivo studies to be hepatoprotective and antihepatotoxic against liver disease induced by alphanaphthylisothiocyanate, $CCl_4$, bromobenzene, and 2-nitropropane.

Both in vivo and human studies have reported that green tea generally inhibits tumors of the liver, esophagus, stomach, small intestine, pancreas, colon, lungs, and breast. In vivo and human trials also showed significant reduction of serum cholesterol and LDL levels and subsequent increases of HDL levels with green tea intake. Green tea has also been found to be active against HIV and the influenza virus. The chemical compounds in green tea block the adhesion of the influenza virus to normal cells.

Caffeine, although frowned upon by diet purists, is a natural substance produced by plants that has actually been found to be a potent antitumor agent and to enhance the cytotoxicity of chemotherapeutic drugs used in treatment of cancer.

**Preparation and Dosage:** Use as tea in prepared tea bags or 1 tsp (5 mL) in 8 ounces (240 mL) water; let steep. Consume as much as desired. A minimum of 4 cups a day is suggested to help prevent cancer. Do not add milk, because it binds to the constituents in green tea and renders them inactive for medicinal purposes.

**Contraindications and Side Effects:** None.

## Decaffeinating Tea

If you do not like caffeine, don't buy a decaffeinated green tea — just let the tea steep longer than 2 minutes. More tannins in the tea come out the longer it steeps; they then bind to the caffeine molecules, making them unusable by your body.

## SPIRULINA *(Spirulina platensis)*

**Family:** Oscillatoriaceae.

**Part used:** Spirulina, although called an algae, is actually spiraled cyanobacteria, one of the most ancient forms of life on Earth. The whole organism is used.

**Collection and habitat:** Spirulina grows wild on ponds and lakes throughout the world. It was one of the food staples (actually the primary protein source) of both the Maya and Aztecs. It is usually commercially grown and harvested and then dried for use. It is commonly called blue-green algae.

**Actions:** Antioxidant, nutrient, tumor inhibitor, antiviral, immunostimulant, vulnerary, detoxifier, tonic.

**Functions in liver disease:** Hepatoprotective, antihepatotoxic, antitumor, nutrient (source of easily digestible proteins, minerals, amino acids, and vitamins). Allows the liver to take in nutrients with little work. Stimulates macrophage and T-cell production and activity. Lowers serum cholesterol and LDL levels. Contains thyroxine precursors and thus helps thyroid function. Helps detoxify the blood, easing the load on the liver. Provides the amino acids necessary for glutathione production.

### About Spirulina

Spirulina is an exceptionally potent nutrient substance that has shown strong activity in many areas. It is the source of one of the most easily digestible forms of protein; it is 85 percent protein, compared with 20 percent in beef. It contains all the essential amino acids and most of the nonessential ones. In addition, it is extremely high in vitamins and minerals.

Spirulina has been found to he hepatoprotective and antihepatotoxic in several in vivo studies, protecting the liver against $CCl_4$-induced hepatotoxicity. Spirulina also contains phycocyanin, a blue-pigment biliprotein that has been shown in scientific studies to inhibit formation of cancer cell colonies.

**Preparation and Dosage:** 1–2 tsp (5–10 mL) powdered spirulina per day, more for chronic or acute disease. Suggested minimum dosage for hepatitis is 4 tsp (20 mL) per day. Consume as much as desired; it may be used as the primary protein source in the diet.

**Contraindications and Side Effects:** None noted.

## THE TEN-WEEK LOW-FAT CLEANSING DIET

Shifting your diet for 2 to 3 months according to the following plan will give your liver a rest and allow much more rapid recovery from liver disease and hepatitis. Many people with hepatitis C lose weight; if this is a problem for you, be sure to include enough protein and oils in your meals when on any low-fat diet. Make sure you include a protein (see Meat on page 92) 1 to 2 times per week. Eat sardines and mackerel as a snack at least once per week, and eat chlorella and spirulina to ensure that you are receiving enough protein in a form your liver can easily use.

1. Drink 6–8 glasses of water every day. Do not use tap water.
2. Eliminate all dairy products, eggs, and sweets.
3. Eat whole grains (brown rice, millet, barley, oats, quinoa, etc.), beans, lightly steamed vegetables, fruit, and meat 1–2 times per week (see pages 90–93). Nuts and seeds contain large amounts of fat and should be eliminated (except for milk thistle seeds). Tempeh and tofu are okay. Do not cook any grains with oil.

**4.** Use only olive oil for cooking. It is naturally antibiotic and will not go rancid. Use no more than 3 tbs (45 mL) of oil per day. Do not use margarine of any kind. You may use butter on food (that is, do not cook or heat the butter).

**5.** Drink all the fresh vegetable juices you like. Fruit juices are great, and fresh-squeezed is preferred. Use only organic apple juice.

**6.** Do not use salt. Use tamari, soy, and any other spices you like, especially ones from the list.

**7.** The only caffeine source should be green tea. Alcohol should be limited to one glass of wine per day or one naturally fermented beer from the list on page 92.

**8.** Eat fruits first and alone. They digest rapidly and, when eaten with other foods, are held in the stomach, where they can cause gas and intestinal problems.

**9.** Do not eat any fried foods.

### List of Recommended Foods for the Cleansing Diet

The following list of foods for the cleansing diet includes foods that will put minimum stress on your liver. In many instances, these foods contain substances that are specific for the healing of liver disease and hepatitis. And, in most instances, they actually taste good.

**Fruits.** Use any fruits you wish. You might want to consider oranges, peaches, and peach kernels. Both sweet and bitter oranges have been found to be strongly hepatoprotective and antihepatotoxic. One of the benefits from oranges (or any citrus fruit) is that the peel is extremely good for helping with the nausea that so often accompanies hepatitis. Eat a little of the peel as often as desired.

Peaches, peach kernels, and peach leaves *(Prunus persica)* have been found to accelerate hepatic regeneration by improving circulation. Peach kernels protect against $CCl_4$-induced chronic hepatitis in vivo.

**Vegetables.** All of the vegetables in the list on page 91 are acceptable. Besides garlic, beets, and artichokes, other vegetables that are especially good for hepatitis and liver disease are dandelion greens, raw carrots and carrot juice, asparagus, burdock, beet greens, and rhubarb. In one study, rhubarb *(Rheum officinale)* at a single dose of 50 g (1.8 oz) per person was effectively used to treat 80 patients with acute icteric hepatitis. (Excessive

## RECOMMENDED VEGETABLES

| | | | |
|---|---|---|---|
| Acorn squash | Cooked carrots | Parsnips | String beans |
| Artichoke | Corn | Potatoes | Summer squash |
| Asparagus | Cucumber | Pumpkins | Sweet potatoes |
| Beets | Daikon | Raw carrots | Swiss chard |
| Broccoli | Daikon greens | Red leafy lettuce | Tomatoes |
| Brussels sprouts | Dandelion | Red radish | Turnip greens |
| Burdock | Eggplant | Rhubarb | Turnips |
| Butternut squash | Jicama | Romaine lettuce | Watercress |
| Cabbage | Kale | Rutabaga | Zucchini |
| Cauliflower | Mustards | Snow peas | |
| Celery | Onion | Spinach | |
| Collards | Parsley | Sprouts, all | |

carrot juice intake should be avoided because it can, over time, cause cirrhosis itself. However, one 16-ounce [30 mL] glass per day is fine.)

**Oil.** Use only olive oil. You might want to consider eating a tin of sardines or mackerel once a week because these fish are exceptionally high in omega-3 fatty acids, which are very good for you.

**Salad dressing.** Use herbed vinegar made with champagne, wine, or fruit vinegars only.

**Seasonings.** Any seasoning but salt is acceptable. Those especially good are cumin, celery seed, and fennel seed. All three have shown strong liver-regeneration stimulation in scientific studies. Turmeric is also good, and clinical trials in humans have shown that basil (*Ocimum sanctum*) and the sages (*Salvia* spp.) have strong hepatoprotective activity.

**Beverages.** Following are the guidelines for what you can drink:

1. Filtered or artesian spring water. Do not use distilled water.
2. Any fruit and vegetable juices. However, avoid all frozen concentrated juices.

3. Herbal teas, especially ginger, peppermint, chamomile, licorice, green, and boneset teas.
4. Beers: Belgian lambic ales, Chimay ale, any beers fermented in the bottles. The label will call it "bottle-conditioned" (there aren't very many, although a good home brew store or beer store will have a good selection). Up to 1 per day.
5. Any wines, up to 1 glass per day.

---

## Alcohol Use

In moderation, alcohol is quite good for people and is a naturally occurring substance produced by plants. In liver disease, however, one of the problems is that alcohol is a liver stimulant (that is, it increases liver activity). In chronic hepatitis, the liver is already overstimulated. Alcohol intake should be limited until the liver is restored to health. (The alcohol in herbal tinctures is present in small quantities and doesn't seem problematic in clinical practice.) There is some indication that in the presence of any quantity of alcohol (more than one glass of wine), HCV can mutate faster and become more active.

Furthermore, alcohol seems to increase sleep disorders, especially if consumed in the evening before bed. Sleep arrives nicely, but at 3:00 A.M. the liver wakes you up and prompts thoughts about all the evils of the world. So, alcohol intake should be lessened for the duration of the disease. Alcohol should be limited to naturally occurring fermentations: wine and beer. No more than one or, at most, two glasses per day. No distilled alcohol should be consumed. Only beers that are natural fermentations and are carbonated in the bottle should be consumed. Belgian lambics, which taste like a slightly sour chardonnay, are highly recommended. They are fermented with several yeasts, including lactobacillus, which give the beverages their distinctive taste. Lactobacilli are extremely good to consume during hepatitis and liver disease.

---

**Meat.** Eat wild meats only, such as elk, venison, and fish from the sea. Do not eat salmon unless you are positive it is wild. Most salmon are grown in ocean pens and are heavily dosed with antibiotics and hormones. Mackerel and sardines are especially good as sources of omega-3 fatty acids. Whey protein, which you can buy in health food stores, is a good substance to add to the diet because it is high in glutamine precursors. Spirulina and chlorella are also two excellent sources of protein that are exceptionally easy on the liver.

**Bread.** Use the healthiest bread you can find. Sprouted grain breads are recommended.

**Cooking.** Use only stainless steel, enameled, or earthenware cooking utensils. Never use aluminum because it will react chemically with the food.

**Sweets.** Use pure maple syrup or organic wildflower honey. Maple syrup contains enough essential ingredients that you could live on it for extended periods. It supplies nearly all the essential vitamins and minerals necessary for health.

# RECIPES FOR THE CLEANSING DIET

It is best to establish a routine for meals. Cook a large pot of grain of your choice or a large pot of soup and keep it in the refrigerator. Then, if you get hungry, there is always something available.

Following is a sample menu for 1 day's worth of meals. You may eat as much as you wish all through the day. Fruit is a good item to have available to eat whenever you feel hungry and to use as a snack food. It is helpful to get a good vegetarian cookbook and plan out a week's meals.

**Breakfast:** Green tea, oatmeal with raisins and maple syrup *or* 16 ounces (480 mL) juiced carrots and beets (⅔ carrots, ⅓ beets), toast with orange marmalade and butter.

**Lunch:** Hepatitis Soup (see page 95), bread and butter, green tea *or* steamed vegetables and astragalus rice, green tea.

**Dinner:** Shark baked in foil with lemon, onion, and celery seed. Mixed green dandelion salad with greek olives, herb vinegar, and olive oil. Cooked beet greens. Belgian lambic ale.

**Desserts and Snacks:** Crystallized ginger slices, fruit.

## Helpful Tips on the Diet Experience

1. It is normal to feel a sensation usually described as hunger when you are on a low-fat diet, no matter how much you eat. This sensation is the feeling that accompanies your body's consumption of its stores of fat.

**2.** You may feel light-headed; this is also normal.

**3.** Since eating is such a social event, it is normal to feel left out when others go out to eat. Go with them and get them to try a good health food restaurant. Order food that comes from this list and is light on oils. A caution about Mexican food: Cheese and sour cream are often put on these otherwise perfect dishes; ask about this when you order.

**4.** When others order alcohol and you also wish to drink, order sparkling water with lime served in a champagne glass, or order a light wine (one glass) or a beer from the list.

**5.** Many emotional issues may arise during any change in eating, especially when the body is using up its store of fat. Remember that this is normal, and make no major life decisions during this time. Remember that you are only doing this for 10 weeks, and it will pass.

## SOME OF THE BEST LIVER FOODS

**Artichoke.** Artichoke is a wonderful healing food for the liver and gallbladder, and it counteracts cholestasis. According to in vivo and in vitro studies, it is highly hepatoprotective and antihepatotoxic against liver damage induced by $CCl_4$, chloroform, chlorinated hydrocarbon, and ethanol. In animals with portions of their liver removed, the liver rapidly regenerated when the animals received artichoke in their diet. Artichoke also reversed fatty degeneration of the liver in several in vivo studies. Eat as many artichoke hearts and steamed artichokes as you want.

**Beets.** Beets contain betane, also found in milk thistle seed, which is a strong hepatoprotector and hepatoregenerator itself. Some physicians in Europe have successfully used beets alone to treat serious liver disease. Beets are also strongly choleretic and dramatically increase bile production and flow. Consume one beet per day, juiced or steamed. Beets are contraindicated in patients with obstructed bile duct.

**Garlic.** Garlic is strongly protective of the liver and helps inactivate liver toxins. It has been found in vivo and in vitro to protect against hepatotoxicity caused by $CCl_4$, allyl alcohol, bromobenzene, galactosamine, and aflatoxin B1. It decreases triglyceride levels and hepatic lipid content. Garlic also strongly enhances immune functioning and regulates cholesterol and lipid levels in the blood. Eat liberally.

## Hepatitis Soup

*Here is a great soup for liver disease and hepatitis. It will strengthen and tonify the immune system as well as provide direct healing for the liver itself.*

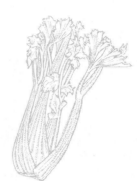

8 cups water
1 tbs (15 mL) olive oil
1 large onion, diced
2 large beets, diced
3–4 tomatoes, diced
1 bulb garlic, minced
1–1½ inch piece of ginger root,
    peeled and finely chopped
1 cup sliced burdock roots
1 bunch sliced kale or beet greens
5 slices dried astragalus root
    (removed when done)
2 cups shiitake mushrooms (fresh or
    reconstituted)
1 whole reishi mushroom (removed
    when done)
½–1 cup spirulina
celery seed, turmeric, and tamari to taste

Combine water and all ingredients in a large pot, bring to a boil, and reduce heat. Simmer for 2–3 hours until vegetables are soft. Season to taste with celery seed, tamari, turmeric. Eat as desired throughout the day.

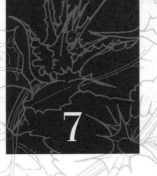

# THE COMPLETE HCV PROTOCOL

B ecause each person actually has a slightly different form of HCV, and because each person's physical health and constitution are slightly different, the herbal protocol for each person should be slightly different. Herbal protocols can be refined for each person by a good herbalist (see Resources).

The following protocol (given as two options) is a good general one for chronic hepatitis C. There are a lot of herbs and supplements to take; most practitioners I have spoken with have found (as I discovered in my own case) that a complex protocol with large quantities of many herbs is necessary for an extended period (usually 6 months to a year). Chronic hepatitis C takes a long time in the building, and the damage the disease causes is slow and deep. It takes a lot of work to reverse it, but that sure beats liver transplantation.

## Protocol Parts

Some of the specific symptoms that hepatitis C causes and herbs that may help alleviate them are covered later in this chapter, after discussion of the protocol itself. Protocol 1 has four elements: liver herbs, immune herbs, nutritional supplements, and diet change. Massage is a suggested fifth element.

96

Although blood readings may change in as little as 2 or 3 months, the protocol should be followed for at least 6 months to a year. HCV is a stealth virus — it also lives in the lymph system and cerebrospinal fluid. Your overall sense of health, not blood tests alone, should guide you.

If any adverse reactions appear, you should 1) stop the protocol, and 2) consult a qualified health care professional.

## HEPATITIS PROTOCOL — OPTION 1

For maximum effect, the following liver and immune herbs are suggested. I have broken down the liver herb regimen into five parts: 1) milk thistle; 2) turmeric paste balls; 3) reishi syrup decoction; 4) dandelion/burdock combination; and 5) capsules of bupleurum, picrorhiza, and phyllanthus.

The immune regimen is broken down into three parts: two different tincture combinations, and capsules of ashwagandha, codonopsis, and tienchi ginseng.

> **Measurement Conversions to Know**
>
> 30 drops = ¼ tsp = 1.25 mL
> ½ tsp = 2.5 mL
> 1 tsp = 5 mL
> 3 tsp = 1 tbl
> 1 tbl = 15 mL
> 2 tbl = 1 ounce
> 1 ounce = 30 mL

### Liver Herbs

**Part 1.** Milk thistle; choose one of the following three options: 1) standardized tincture (store purchased), standardized to 140 mg silybum flavinoids, 25 drops 3 times per day; 2) nonstandardized tincture, ½ tsp (2.5 mL) 3 times per day; 3) powdered seed, 3 tbl (45 mL) per day.

**Part 2.** Turmeric paste balls (about the size of a marble): 4 per day.

**Part 3.** Reishi syrup: 3.5 ounces (105 mL) 3 times per day. (May substitute 2–4 tsp [10–20 mL] tincture 3 times per day or 3 "00" capsules 3 times per day).

**Part 4.** Combine equal parts dandelion and burdock root tinctures, take 1 tsp (5 mL) 3 times per day. (May be taken instead as capsules: burdock, 2–3 capsules [1–1.5 g] 3 times per day; dandelion, 4–5 capsules [2–2.5 g] 3 times per day).

**Part 5.** 2 "00" capsules each of bupleurum, picrorhiza, and phyllanthus 3 times per day.

### Immune Herbs

**Part 1.** Combine equal parts of astragalus, Siberian ginseng, and panax ginseng tinctures; take ½ tsp (75 drops, 2.5 mL) 3 times per day.
**Part 2.** Combine equal parts licorice, red root, and schizandra tinctures; take ½ tsp (75 drops, 2.5 mL) 3 times per day.
**Part 3.** 2 "00" capsules each of ashwagandha, codonopsis, and tienchi ginseng 3 times per day.

### Nutritional Supplements

**1.** 50 mg chelated zinc once per day.
**2.** 800 mg vitamin E once per day.
**3.** Comprehensive B vitamin complex once per day.
**4.** 4 g vitamin C as C salts, ⅓ tsp 3 times per day.
**5.** 200 mg alpha-lipoic acid 3 times per day.
**6.** *N*-acetylcysteine, 600 mg 3 times per day; take with food.

### Diet

Follow recommendations in chapter 6. In general, reduce fat and alcohol intake; increase vegetable and grain intake; use foods that will reduce work load on the liver; use foods known to have positive effect on the liver and immune system.

### Massage

A Swedish full-body massage once a week is highly recommended.

## HEPATITIS PROTOCOL — OPTION 2

I got tired of taking so many separate supplements and now use a pre-mixed formula developed by Dry Creek Herb Farm in Auburn, California (see Resources). Although several different formulas are available from Dry Creek, the one I take contains milk thistle, dandelion, burdock, bupleurum, phyllanthus, turmeric, licorice, astragalus,

Siberian ginseng, ashwagandha, chlorella, spirulina, and bladderwrack. All are in powder form.

The premixed formula may be taken as ⅙ cup powder 3 times per day, ¼ cup powder 2 times per day, or ½ cup powder once per day blended in juice. I use ½ cup of the combined powder blended in 12 ounces (360 mL) apple juice and water (in equal parts) just before bed each evening. It's a bit gritty but isn't that awful-tasting once you get used to it. It is much more convenient to use than the extensive number of capsules and tinctures outlined in Hepatitis Protocol — Option 1.

In addition to the premixed formula, I also take a tincture of panax ginseng and tienchi ginseng (full dropper, 30 drops or 1.25 mL) 2 times per day; the same amount of schizandra tincture 2 times per day; and, at 4:00 P.M. each day, a reishi syrup decoction to which I add 1 tbl boldo leaf during the decoction process. I take the complete list of nutritional supplements outlined in Option 1, as well. The tinctures and supplements are taken upon rising in the morning and just before bed. The diet and massage recommendations should be part of this protocol, too.

## HERBS FOR SPECIFIC SYMPTOMS

There are a number of specific and unique symptoms that people experience when they have hepatitis. Some of these are common to nearly everyone with HCV; others occur irregularly. The following list covers most of the symptoms that HCV can cause and the herbs that can help alleviate them.

**Abdominal bloating, fluid retention, puffy face:** Dandelion leaf, burdock seed, and (for puffy face) codonopsis.

**Adverse reactions to alcohol:** Limit or eliminate alcohol in diet.

**Aversion to fatty foods:** This will improve as the herbal protocol is followed, but your body is trying to tell you something. Limit fat intake to 3 tbl (45 mL) fats/oils per day.

**Blood sugar disorders:** Dandelion root, devil's club root bark (*Oplopanax horridum*), 10–40 drops of tincture up to 3 times per day, milk thistle, panax ginseng.

**Chest pains, palpitations:** Motherwort (*Leonarus cardiaca*), 30–60 drops up to 4 times per day; strong tea, 2–4 ounces (50–120 mL) as desired; baical skullcap; reishi.

**Chronic fatigue, sudden attacks of exhaustion, weakness:** Support good sleep as much as possible. Keep up a good regimen of immune herbs and foods. For the short-term, 16 ounces fresh beet/carrot juice (⅓ : ⅔ proportion), green tea (as much as desired), panax ginseng, codonopsis, massage. *Note:* Do not take ginseng or green tea before bed because they may interfere with sleep.

**Cirrhosis:** Milk thistle, picrorhiza, reishi, turmeric.

**Depression, mood swings, seasonal affective disorder:** Weekly massage. St.-John's-wort *(Hypericum perfoliatum)* tincture of fresh plant, 20–30 drops up to 3 times per day or standard capsules from a store (follow directions on the package); ashwagandha, schizandra, Siberian ginseng.

**Diarrhea:** Blackberry leaf *(Rubus villosus)* or raspberry leaf *(Rubus idaeus)* tea, as much as desired; 1 tsp (5 mL) leaf to 1 cup water, steep 15 minutes.

**Dizziness:** Herbal hepatitis protocol, ginkgo, codonopsis.

**Flulike illness, intermittent chills and fever:** Boneset, echinacea, baical skullcap, bupleurum, picrorhiza, turmeric.

**Frequent urination:** Mullein root (*Verbascum* spp., to increase sphincter control), 2–3 ounces (15–45 mL) strong decoction 2–3 times per day or 30–50 drops in tincture 2 times per day; no water or liquids before bed.

**Indigestion/nausea:** A small slice of orange, lemon, or lime peel eaten fresh as needed will almost always work. The relief lasts from 5 minutes to days. Crystallized ginger root as needed. Of lesser benefit but still worthwhile, picrorhiza, gentian *(Gentiana lutea),* 5–20 drops before meals or as needed.

**Irregular menses, premenstrual syndrome:** Dong quai *(Angelica sinensis),* 5–20 drops tincture up to 3 times per day; black cohosh *(Cimifuga racemosa),* 10–25 drops up to 3 times per day; vitex *(Vitex agnus-castus)* in the absence of depression, 30–60 drops each morning. These will help more over a period of several months.

**Irritability:** Will improve with herbal protocol over time. Short-term: baical skullcap, pasque flower *(Anemone pusitilla),* 5–10 drops not more than once each hour (may cause nausea); motherwort, 30–60 drops up to 4 times per day, massage.

**High cholesterol:** Burdock, dandelion, milk thistle, turmeric, garlic.

**Joint pain:** Reishi, turmeric, ashwagandha.

**Liver cancer:** Burdock, turmeric, reishi, astragalus, Siberian ginseng, panax ginseng. *Note:* I highly recommend Donald Yance's book, *Herbal Medicine, Healing & Cancer.*

**Loss of appetite:** Bupleurum, milk thistle, phyllanthus, codonopsis.

**Low libido:** Panax or Siberian ginseng (depending on age), ginger, ashwagandha, better sleep, immune protocol, herbal hepatitis protocol, massage.

**Mental fatigue, cognitive dysfunction, brain fog, attention deficit disorder:** Reishi, ginkgo *(Ginkgo biloba)*, 30–60 drops up to 3 times per day, Siberian ginseng, ashwagandha, panax ginseng, green tea, massage.

**Numbness in extremities:** Herbal hepatitis protocol, better sleep, massage, panax ginseng (over time), ginger.

**Skin problems (itchy skin, skin eruptions, itching around orifices: eyes, nose, ears, rectum):** Burdock, dandelion, milk thistle, bupleurum (especially for itching), phyllanthus. If especially bad, add ½ tsp (2.5 mL), 3 times per day, of equal-part tincture of fresh nettles *(Urtica dioica)* and fresh red clover blossoms *(Trifolium pratense).*

**Sleep disorders (vivid dreams, night sweats, irregular and poor sleep quality, feeling tired after sleep):** These problems take awhile to improve; they will get better as the herbal protocol is followed. Some things that will help in the meantime are weekly massage and eating carbohydrates 30 minutes to 1 hour before bedtime (this will automatically make you more drowsy). Never eat meat in the evening or drink more than one glass of wine. Never consume any foods that are high in preservatives before bedtime.

In other words, ease the stress on the liver so that it works less hard while you sleep. In this instance, alcohol seems to aggravate sleep disorders. Herbs that may help are reishi, baical skullcap, and boldo (all of which should specifically be included in the herbal regimen if sleep disorders are a problem). Of limited benefit may be ½ ounce (3 tsp, 15 mL) of a tincture composed of equal parts motherwort *(Leonarus cardiaca)* and wood betony *(Pedicularis* spp.) used in water or juice just before bed. Valerian and hops should be avoided because they both tend to increase depression and, at least in hepatitis, do not seem to work as well as the motherwort/wood betony combination.

**Stabbing pains in the liver region:** Boldo, reishi, and, to a limited extent, Culver's root *(Leptandra virginica)*, 3–10 drops tincture as needed. Will work only for a limited time. Fringetree bark *(Chionanthus virginica)*, 20–40 drops as desired. Will help occasionally.

**Swellings under armpits, in groin, around neck:** Red root.

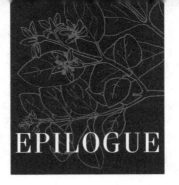

# EPILOGUE

# AGGRESSIVE SYMBIONTS: THE SPECTER OF EMERGING VIRUSES

In the summer of 1999, a mysterious virus appeared in New York City. The virus was carried by a common mosquito, and by the time it had run its course 7 people were dead and 52 were hospitalized. New York and the nation were riveted, and afraid. The virus, originally thought to be St. Louis encephalitis, was discovered to be the West Nile virus, a mosquito-borne virus never known to exist in the western hemisphere.

In recent years, stories of such viral incursions into the human species, sometimes from strange-sounding viruses such as Ebola Zaire and Marburg (and now HCV), have become common. It is rare that a month goes by without a news article about them, although of course these pale in comparison to the most famous of new viruses, HIV, the cause of AIDS, which is in the news daily. Such reports, and others tracking the increasing resistance of bacteria to antibiotics, make clear that the microbial world is changing, that new diseases are flourishing, and that these diseases are encroaching on the human sphere with increasing frequency. Emerging viruses promise to change the nature of disease and its treatment in the coming decades: Diseases long thought conquered, or, even more grimly, completely unknown, are now a part of our lives and futures.

# THE FUNCTION OF VIRUSES

Sometimes awake and replicating, sometimes asleep and hibernating, there are literally millions of kinds of viruses. Most are found in the rain forests. Although researchers have identified about 4000 viruses, it is estimated that each of the 30 million species of life on Earth has at least one virus living in compatible symbiosis within it. But there can be more than one; some caterpillars have been found with 60 different viruses inside them. The number of viruses that we can encounter as a species is simply incredible. In fact, given their number, they very rarely cause disease. Of the millions of viruses, only about 150 are known to cause human disease, while another 400 or so could cause human disease should they "jump species" into us. In fact, the function of viruses is quite different from the role of lurking, predatory, uncaring disease pathogens they have been shaped to be in modern imagination. They, like bacteria, are necessary for life on Earth.

> "Viruses are no more 'germs' and 'enemies' than are bacteria or human cells."
>
> — LYNN MARGULIS, PhD,
> SYMBIOTIC PLANET: A NEW
> LOOK AT EVOLUTION

## Symbiogenesis

Substantial evidence suggests that all complex forms of life on Earth have evolved through what is now being called *symbiogenesis.* In symbiogenesis, two aggressive bacteria come together and, instead of one killing the other, merge to form a uniquely different third organism that contains the genetic structure of both. Over long aeons, this process of mutual collaboration has resulted in very complex arrangements, such as those that form the human body. In fact, using gene analysis, researchers such as Lynn Margulis have shown that the mitochondria and white blood cells in the human body are in fact former free-living bacteria that in ages past formed a symbiosis with what we now recognize as us.

We are, in fact, formed of the very bacteria that we have been taught to fear, that we have been trying to kill off since the invention of antibiotics. As scientists are now grimly learning, we cannot kill off the bacteria that cause disease without also killing off all life on Earth. For many of the same reasons, we cannot kill off the viruses that cause disease. Viruses, like bacteria, play an essential part in the coevolution of all life on Earth. We are our viruses as well as our bacteria.

## THE DISCOVERY OF VIRUSES

Viruses were discovered as a separate entity in 1885, when several researchers found that the organism that causes tobacco mosaic disease in tobacco plants was not visible under a microscope and that it could pass through the finest porcelain filters. One of the men, Martinus Willem Beijerinck, called it a "contagious living fluid," but eventually all such organisms were given the broad Latin name of *virus*, which simply means "poison."

## THE VIRAL WORLD

Viruses inhabit a unique ecological niche: the landscape of the genome, of DNA and RNA. Viruses not only speak the language of genes but also write that language. Viruses possess an incredible ability: They can snip off parts of DNA that they encounter and weave it into their own structure. They can also take snippets they carry inside them and weave them into the DNA of other organisms they encounter. In fact, one of their main functions is to intermingle the genetic structure of all life on Earth. They have been doing this for a long, long time, and we have not been exempt from it.

For instance, people who have a genetic marker known as HLA-B27 have a tendency to get a disease called ankylosing spondylitis, a severe form of arthritis. No one knew why until researches realized that the HLA-B27 genetic marker is identical to a section of the DNA of the *Klebsiella pneumoniae* bacterium. In some ancient time, a virus

"This landscape, the landscape of the genome, is the world a virus, in human terms, might call home. No other form of life inhabits this extraordinary ecological niche. And in the way of all life, the virus changes the landscape, just as the landscape molds the virus."

— FRANK RYAN, MD

encountered a *K. pneumoniae* bacterium and snipped off a bit of DNA, interweaving it with its own. Later, inside a human, it interwove that snippet with the DNA of a nucleus destined to be an egg or sperm. Specifically, the *Klebsiella* DNA was interwoven with the genes that carry instructions for forming ligaments and tendons. Thus, this tiny part of a bacterium began to pass down through human generations, from one child to the next. And from time to time, one of those descendants would actually become infected with *K. pneumoniae*. Their immune system would gear up, produce antibodies to the bacteria, and clear it from the system.

But here is where the problem begins. There are still some *K. pneumoniae* genes in the body, in the nucleus of the cells of the ligaments and tendons throughout the body. The antibodies, seeking *K. pneumoniae*, notice the HLA-B27 genetic marker, swarm to the ligaments and tendons, and attack them, causing ankylosing spondylitis.

> "From kittens to fireflies to weeds, into the sea and back again, the viruses wander without aim, snipping off a piece of heredity here, depositing it there, exchanging the code of life like bits of gossip passed over a backyard fence. . . . Viruses are the worst gossips in the world."
>
> — CHARLES PELLEGRINO, PhD, COAUTHOR OF *CHRONIC FATIGUE SYNDROME*

## Viral Jumping

Normally, viruses, like bacteria, establish symbiosis with other life-forms with which they coevolve. Their host organisms provide a home to them and, like coevolutionary bacteria, viruses provide things for their hosts. One of the provided benefits is gene reassortment, which helps the organism adapt and evolve at a much faster rate than the slow aeons of change that standard evolutionary theory predicts.

In a healthy symbiosis, a virus never kills off its host, for then it will either go dormant or die, depending on its nature. And viruses, like all life, have the urge to survive and reproduce. A virus causes disease only when it jumps from a coevolved host into a new species, and viruses jump species only if their habitat is disturbed.

Physicians in Brazil have noticed that as new immigrants enter the rain forest to cut trees, they begin to fall ill with diseases no one has seen before. In fact, a whole new group of viruses (group C) have emerged in the human species in Brazil, viruses that have lived in peace in the rain forest for millennia. This same story is being played out all over the globe and has caused a rethinking of what scientists thought they knew about viruses.

### Disturbing the Anthill

Virologists have discovered that when a balanced symbiotic virus is disturbed, it tends to jump species. They have termed this tendency *aggressive symbiosis*.

There are approximately 4000 mammal species on Earth (in contrast, there are 750,000 insect species). Of those mammal species, about 2000 are rodents and 1000 are bats. Most of the viruses that jump species and infect people (although definitely not all) come from rodents, bats, and primates. Hantavirus, the mysterious virus that killed many Navajo in the American Southwest a few years ago, is spread in mouse feces. One of the properties of viruses as aggressive symbiotic organisms is that they pour out of their symbiotic host into the environment, often in feces or urine. This "salts" the environment with dormant virus particles so that any encroaching species will immediately come into contact with them. With hantavirus, many people acquired the virus and ultimately died simply because they swept their floors and stirred up this "viral salt." A unique mouse population in the area had increased in response to many broad environmental factors, including global warming. This allowed the development of a pathogen that had previously been unknown in humans in the Americas.

In another example, a squirrel monkey in the Amazonian rain forest has a balanced coevolutionary symbiosis with a virus, herpesvirus saimiri. Even if the monkey's immune system is artificially suppressed, the virus will cause it no harm. The entire ecoregion the monkeys inhabit is liberally salted with the virus through urine and feces excretion. If a competing primate, the marmoset monkey (whose range occasionally crosses that of the squirrel monkey), moves into the squirrel

> "The fact that we have opposable thumbs, know how to use vacuum cleaners, and listen to opera simply doesn't matter to viruses."
>
> —C. J. Peters, MD, Chief of Special Pathogens at the Centers for Disease Control and Prevention

monkey territory, the virus immediately jumps. It causes a tremendously quick fulminating cancer of the lymphatic system in marmoset monkeys. The invading monkeys die off, and the squirrel monkeys, and their ecosystem, are left undisturbed.

Epstein-Barr virus, the smallpox virus, and many of the emerging South American viruses have jumped from rodent species. Measles jumped into humans from wild cattle or ungulates that were domesticated 5000 to 6000 years ago. Smallpox still contains long gene sequences of mouse DNA. As Egyptians felled forests and planted more and more land to grain, one type of mouse (a mouse that possessed smallpox as an evolutionary symbiont), normally restricted to small numbers in a localized ecoregion, was permitted to surge out of its natural habitat and explosively expand its population. In the process, smallpox virus was liberally salted into the growing fields of grain and storage silos. From there it jumped into humans.

## WHERE DID SMALLPOX GO?

The smallpox virus was considered eradicated in 1977, and vaccination programs ceased in 1980. Unfortunately, secret stockpiles of the virus were kept, its virulence increased through accelerating normal viral mutation in biological weapons laboratories throughout the Soviet Union. At the breakup of that country, many of these supplies of smallpox, now estimated at 200 tons of live virus, simply disappeared.

Humans now have the same immunity to smallpox that they did when it entered the species some 5000 years ago: none. No reliable supplies of vaccine exist. And oddly enough, given the vaccine's simplicity, no company in the world can make it. Like all viruses, smallpox didn't disappear; it has simply gone into a new and unique form of hibernation until conditions become right for its reemergence.

This kind of aggressive symbiosis is not uncommon in nature. Many ant species live in the same kind of symbiosis with plants. In exchange, the plants provide special nutrients for them. If a hungry herbivore moves in and begins to eat the plant, the ants swarm out and bite and sting its nose and tongue until it leaves. Viral researcher Stefan Pattyn comments that the viral/host cycle is like such a colony of ants that has been living in the wilderness for aeons. "Human intrusion into the local ecology causes the anthill to be destroyed. The ants swarm out and attack." Richard Preston, who wrote the best-selling book *The Hot Zone,* is more blunt, and chilling.

> *The AIDS virus and other emerging viruses are surviving the wreck of the tropical biosphere because they can mutate faster than any changes taking place in their ecosystems. They must be good at escaping trouble, if some of them have been around for four billion years. I tend to think of rats leaving a sinking ship. . . . AIDS is the revenge of the rain forest. It is only the first act of the revenge.*

It turns out that HIV, the virus that causes AIDS, came out of the rain forests in Africa, where it lives in monkeys in a balanced symbiosis. Two things brought HIV out of hiding and into the modern human world: human encroachment into and devastation of jungle habitat, and modern medicine. Modern medicine plays a dual role in the emergence of HIV. The first is medical technology itself: blood transfusions, needles, surgeries, and the large numbers of monkeys sought for medical experiments, all of which allow the transmission of the disease into humans. The second is the immunization programs carried out in Africa between 1955 and 1975. Many of the vaccines were made by using kidney cells from monkeys that are symbiotic with HIV. This inserted the virus into thousands of humans when they were vaccinated by health care workers for other diseases. And as they had sex over the course of the next decade, they infected thousands of other people, who infected other thousands, and so on. It is the greatest ecological catastrophe of our time and one of the most pervasive of iatrogenic (medically caused) diseases. Some African countries will lose half their population: all people between the ages of 20 and 45.

Unfortunately, at least 50 other viruses, HCV among them, are emerging into the human species. Some, like the viruses that cause yellow and dengue fevers (close relatives of HCV), have been suppressed for a century or more and are reemerging as a result of modern ecosystem disruption.

# THE INFLUENCE OF HUMAN CULTURE

Changing human cultural patterns also play a strong role in viral emergence. Neither measles nor smallpox could stabilize in human populations until the rise of cities. Researchers have determined that measles needs 500,000 people living in close proximity to remain viable, while smallpox needs 200,000 people living within 14 days' travel of each other. Once these conditions occurred, about 5000 years ago, the respective viruses became regularly infective in humans. (With population densities less than optimal, the virus would kill off the susceptible and simply vanish from the species unless its original habitat were encroached upon again.) Both viruses, to a new immune system, are biosafety level 4 viruses, the most dangerous and deadly.

Our new patterns of life — megacities, airplane travel (all places on Earth are now within 24 hours of each other), technological medicine, monocropping of plants and animals for food, environmental devastation at a level not seen since the dinosaur extinctions 65 million years ago — all have created a situation for the emergence and spread of viruses that are new, frightening, and very hard to treat. Unfortunately, simply viewing viruses as disease pathogens and attempting to eradicate them will not work, any more than eradicating bacteria has worked or can work. Viruses are an intricate part of Earth's ecosystem. Viewing them as common, and essential, members of the life web and approaching treatment from a broad, inclusive, environmental perspective is most likely to solve the problems of viral emergence and to lessen the new problems that short-term solutions create. Part of this perspective means treating diseases such as hepatitis C by treating the whole ecology of the body and viewing the virus as an ally, not an enemy.

When they first enter a new species, viruses are often exceptionally virulent: They are an aggressive symbiont trying to kill off an encroaching life-form. But, over time, viruses begin to establish balance in any species they infect. As the virus and immune system of the new host struggle, there is a tendency for a healthy symbiosis to develop. The virus moves from being an aggressive symbiont of another species to establishing coevolutionary symbiosis with its new one. This often takes hundreds if not thousands of years. Such an event has happened with Epstein-Barr virus, the virus that has been hypothesized to cause chronic fatigue syndrome. This virus is so balanced now that it takes a severely suppressed immune system to allow it to start acting as a disease pathogen.

We cannot kill off the viruses or the bacteria. As with all cultures after a war (this time, the war on disease), perhaps the best approach is to find a way to peacefully coexist. The Cherokee people of North America understood this problem and spoke long ago about the diseases that come from mistreatment of the natural world. Perhaps at this time of incredible world change we can, at last, learn from their wisdom.

*It is told among the Cherokee (and other tribes such as the Creek) that long ago, before there was disease, human beings angered the other members of the life web with which they share the Earth. They had been disrespectful, treating the animals, insects, and plants without kindness or understanding. They were killing them off, trampling their homes, disturbing their families.*

*The insects became tired of it and they decided each to give a disease to human beings. And so, a sickness came out of their body and began to enter the bodies of the human beings. They then sent their king to the animals asking that they also join in each giving a disease to the humans. There was much discussion but in the end it did not take long for them to agree. And there came a sickness out of each of the bodies of the animals that began to enter the bodies of the human beings.*

*Finally, the king of the insects went to the plants and asked them to join in putting an end to the humans. For long and long did the plants think it over, but when the king returned for their answer they replied, "We cannot. For," they said, "the human beings are our children and we must help them even if they are foolish." And then each tree, each shrub and herb, down even to the grasses and mosses, agreed to furnish a remedy for some one of the diseases the insects and animals had given and each plant said: "I shall appear to help man whenever he calls upon me in his need."*

In using plant medicines, in coming to honor the intelligence of viruses and bacteria, we begin restoring our deeply human connection to the life web of Earth and once again finding a way to walk in harmony and balance on this wonderful green planet that is our home.

# APPENDIX 1
## Tests for Hepatitis C and What They Mean

Tests for hepatitis viruses usually focus on blood tests and, sometimes, liver biopsy. This overlooks the fact that HCV may be strongly present in the lymph system or cerebrospinal fluid and absent from the blood at the same time that liver cirrhosis is progressing. The test results should be interpreted in light of a deep knowledge of the disease, the accuracy of the tests themselves, and how you, as the patient, feel about your level of health.

### Antibody Detection Test

In general, this is the first test you will have. It is often done as a part of a general blood screen, many times initiated for some other reason. The test has many names, but it will usually be listed on the laboratory report simply as "hepatitis C AB," meaning hepatitis C antibodies. The result will show up as reactive or nonreactive. "Reactive" means simply that you have at one time been exposed to hepatitis C and your body has formed antibodies to it. It does not indicate the presence of HCV. Usually, many other factors are involved in determining whether or not HCV is present in the body.

In general, the test used will be an ELISA: an enzyme-linked immunosorbent assay. ELISA was first used in 1995; ELISA III, which is much more accurate than the first-generation tests, is now being used. It is still not 100 percent accurate. A more accurate, and more expensive (and hence lesser used), test is RIBA: recombinant immunoblot assay. RIBA III is the best available, but it is still not 100 percent accurate. Both false-positive and false-negative results can occur.

It can take 6 months before your body forms HCV antibodies. If your test results indicate that you are negative for antibodies but you have reason to believe you might still be infected, you should be retested in 6 months.

Some people with HCV have no antibodies and test negative. Some test negative and eventually test positive, and some test positive and are actually negative. It is confusing. The test can be used as a fairly reliable indicator if the result is positive, but you should always look to how some of the other tests turn out. Most especially, you should note how you feel about your health. Remember, you live in your body, your physician does not. Human consciousness is still the most refined instrument of perception known.

### Blood Tests

There is another set of easy tests that will be used to assess your overall liver health; they are usually performed at the same time that blood is tested for HCV antibodies. They are called, in general, liver function tests.

**ALT and AST Tests.** To the confusion of many, the names of these tests have changed, and you may hear and see them referred to under both names. ALT stands for alanine aminotransferase; it is also sometimes called SGPT. AST stands for aspartate aminotransferase and is sometimes called SGOT. Alanine and aspartate aminotransferase are both enzymes present in the liver. When the liver is damaged, cells break down and these enzymes leak into the bloodstream, causing enzyme levels to rise. While AST in the blood can come from other sources, a high ALT level is almost invariably from liver damage. The levels can vary widely in patients with hepatitis, and some people chart the rise and fall over time, feeling that this graph is a good indicator of the health of the liver.

To add confusion, once again, severe liver damage can be present with normal ALT and AST levels, and minor damage can be seen with high levels. One important thing to look for is the ratio of AST to ALT. Some researchers and clinicians feel that a higher level of AST than ALT indicates liver damage or cirrhosis, regardless of the absolute levels of AST or ALT individually. In general, levels lower than 50 IU/L are considered normal, with ALT being higher than AST. These are the two most common indicators referred to in the treatment of people with hepatitis.

**Bilirubin.** Bilirubin, formed from hemoglobin, is filtered by the liver from blood returning from the intestines through the portal vein. Hence, bilirubin in the blood shows that the liver is not functioning well. The higher the level, the worse the liver function. Extremely high levels produce jaundice, a yellowing primarily of the skin, eyes, and back of the throat. Blood levels of bilirubin should be lower than 1.5 mg/dL or 17 ml/L.

**Albumin.** Albumin is a major protein found in the blood. The level of protein (albumin) in the blood directly corresponds to the liver's ability to form proteins. Hence, a low level indicates poor liver function.

**Blood Fat Levels: Cholesterol, HDL, and LDL.** It is common for the presence of these fats to fluctuate during liver disease. Cholesterol and LDL levels may rise; HDL levels may decrease. In advanced liver disease, including cirrhosis, cholesterol, LDL, and HDL levels are significantly lower. High levels of total cholesterol and LDL and low levels of HDL can indicate problems with blood fats and diet in general or be directly related to a poorly functioning liver.

A high LDL level (over 130 mg/dL) is associated with increased incidence of heart attack or stroke; these events are also associated with a low level of HDL (under 35 mg/dL) and a high total serum cholesterol level (over 200 mg/dL).

## Further Tests

If you show the presence of antibodies to HCV, your physician may want to conduct further tests for the presence of HCV itself. Several tests are used for this, including the following ones.

**HCV b-DNA.** HCV b-DNA stands for hepatitis C virus branched DNA. It is sometimes listed as HCV RNA b-DNA. This is the third most common test, primarily because it is fairly cheap. It is not very sensitive and only shows the presence of viral loads above a certain level (350,000 per mL). It is possible to have a negative b-DNA test result and still have hepatitis C. Generally, people who have HCV and test negative on b-DNA are considered to be the best (and sometimes only) candidates for interferon or interferon–ribavirin treatment.

**PCR.** PCR stands for polymerase chain reaction. The test amplifies the virus's nucleic acid many millions of times, bringing it up to "visible" levels. From that "visible" level, the actual levels of the virus in the blood can be mathematically calculated. The test is highly sensitive and can detect viral load levels much smaller than those identified by the b-DNA test, as low as 1000 per mL. The test is expensive and often is not available in smaller cities. The test is highly accurate for certain viral strains and less accurate for others, and it does not detect any virus in the lymph or cerebrospinal fluid should the blood be clear. At present, however, it is the best test for detecting the presence of the virus.

**Liver biopsy.** A liver biopsy is performed by inserting a needle through the abdomen into the liver and removing a small sample of liver tissue. It is considered the best way to determine liver health and can be either an inpatient or outpatient procedure. The procedure and postprocedure observation take 6 to 18 hours. Although considered a minor procedure, there is a chance of complications, with a death rate of 1/10,000 people. Liver biopsy and associated medications have several side effects. You should talk about these candidly with your physician and then base your decision on all the information available.

The liver tissue is examined and a grade is assigned according to the tissue's level of health; the scale ranges from 0 to 6, and the higher the number, the more damage there is to the liver. Many liver specialists insist on liver biopsies and may require more than one.

# APPENDIX 2

## Making and Using Herbal Medicines
## for Hepatitis and the Liver

In general, plants are used as or made into medicines in five ways: by infusing the herb in water (as teas, infusions, decoctions, washes, beers, or steams); by infusing the herb in alcohol or an alcohol and water combination (as tinctures, fluid extracts, and, when diluted, washes or sprays); by transferring the power of the herb to an oil base (salves and oils); by using the plant itself (by eating it whole or using as wound powder, in capsules, by smoking, or by smudging); or by distilling and using the essential oil of the plant. In general, herbs are most useful in hepatitis treatment as teas, in whole form, as food, or as tinctures. Food has already been covered. Let's look at the other three.

There are, of course, other mediums in which herbs can be extracted for use as medicine: vinegar, glycerin, and honey are three good ones. They all extract the medicinal qualities of a plant to differing degrees: Whole herb, water, and alcohol are the strongest, and glycerin and honey are next, followed by vinegar and oil. Glycerin and honey extractions are extremely useful for children because of the sweet taste.

> ### Four Major Forms of Herbal Medicine for Hepatitis
>
> Infusions
> Tinctures
> Whole plant
> Food

## Water Extractions

Water is the primary medium that people have always used for extracting the active components of herbs. It is considered the universal solvent for planet Earth. There are several ways to use water to extract the medicinal actions of herbs. The most common are infusions and decoctions.

## Making Infusions

An infusion is made by immersing an herb in cold or hot, not boiling, water for an extended time. (Basically, a tea is a weak infusion.) The water you use should be the purest you can find, not tap water. Water from rain, water from healthy wells or springs, or distilled water is best. The following guidelines are for hot infusions and will work with most herbs.

> ### When To Make Cold Infusions
>
> Cold infusions are preferable for some herbs. The bitter components of herbs tend to be less water-soluble. Yarrow, for instance, is much less bitter when prepared in cold water. Usually, cold infusions need to steep for much longer periods; each herb is different.

**For leaves:** 1 ounce per quart of water; steep for 4 hours in hot water, tightly covered. Tougher leaves require longer steeping.

**For flowers:** 1 ounce per quart of water; steep for 2 hours in hot water, tightly covered. More fragile flowers require less time.

**For seeds:** 1 ounce per pint of water; steep for 30 minutes in hot water, tightly covered. More fragrant seeds, such as fennel, need less time (15 minutes); rose hips need more time (3–4 hours).

**For barks and roots:** 1 ounce per pint of water; steep for 8 hours in hot water, tightly covered. Some barks, such as slippery elm, need less time (1–2 hours).

Unless you are making a steam, hot infusions should be prepared in tightly covered jars to keep the volatile oils from rising off the infusion as steam. Herbs that have a strong essential oil or perfumy smell when the leaves are crushed are usually high in volatile oils. Quart or pint canning jars are very good because they will not break from heat. In addition, the screw cap allows them to be shaken if desired and keeps any volatile oils from floating off as steam. I usually like to leave them overnight. I prepare them before bed, strain them out the next morning, and drink them throughout the day.

## Making Decoctions

Decoctions, prepared with boiling, can be much more potent than infusions and are generally prepared for use as compresses, enemas, and syrups. The standard pharmaceutical approach to decoctions is 1 ounce of herb per pint of water boiled for 15 minutes and strained when cool; water is then added to bring it back up to 1 pint. I approach it a little differently, as follows.

**1.** Combine 1 ounce herb with 3 cups water in a stainless steel or heat-resistant glass container (never use aluminum).

**2.** Boil slowly and steadily until the liquid is reduced to one-half.

The dosage can range from 1 teaspoon to 1 cup depending on the plant used. If larger amounts of the decoction are desired, the amount of water and herb may be increased. Infusions and decoctions should be kept for no more than 3 days if refrigerated, 1 or 2 days if unrefrigerated.

A decoction can be used to make a compress by simply soaking a sterile bandage in the decoction and then placing it on the appropriate area of the body. It can also be used to make a syrup. You may want to reduce the liquid even further (to two-thirds, as with following recipe) and add honey to taste.

---

### Reishi Syrup Decoction

*This is a powerful way to concentrate the activity of reishi.*

> 5 g reishi
> 1 qt (1 L) water

**To make:** Slowly bring to boil and simmer at lowest boil obtainable for 2 hours, uncovered, until the volume of water is reduced by two-thirds. Cool and strain.

**To use:** Consume the syrup in three equal amounts over the course of 1 day. For acute conditions, the amount consumed can be increased as much as desired.

## Alcohol Extractions

A tincture is made by immersing a fresh or dried plant in either full-strength alcohol or an alcohol and water mixture. Fresh plants naturally contain a certain percentage of water. Alcohol is extractive: It pulls all of the water out of plants into itself. The resulting tincture is a mix of both water and alcohol.

Some people feel that alcohol is completely contraindicated in liver disease. Others have alcohol intolerance or are recovering alcoholics and wish to avoid it. I have found that the amounts of alcohol necessary for the herbal protocol for chronic viral hepatitis are negligible in their effects on the liver. Essentially, you will be consuming a total of ½ ounce of alcohol a day in three doses over 12 to 16 hours. This is not very much, actually. The alcohol also facilitates the absorption of the herbs into the system. If you wish to completely avoid alcohol, you may make your tinctures as glycerites or take the herbs in whole form.

## Tincturing Fresh Herbs

Fresh leafy plants may be chopped or left whole before they are placed into the alcohol, or they can be pureed with the alcohol in a blender. Fresh roots should be ground with the alcohol in a blender into a pulpy mush. Making a tincture using fresh plant matter requires just a few simple steps, as follows.

**1.** In a Mason jar, combine the fresh plant material with 190-proof alcohol (95 percent alcohol), in a ratio of 1 part plant to 2 parts alcohol. (For example, if you had 3 ounces [dry measure] of fresh echinacea flower heads, this amount would be combined with 6 ounces [liquid measure] of 190-proof alcohol.)

**2.** Seal the jar well and store out of the sun for 2 weeks, shaking the jar daily.

**3.** At the end of 2 weeks, decant (strain) the herb through a piece of muslin or cheesecloth, squeezing the herb until as dry as possible to extract all the valuable liquid (an herb or wine press is good for this). Store the resulting liquid in amber bottles that are well labeled with the name of the plant.

## Tincturing Dried Plants

With fresh plant tinctures, you can generally get out about as much liquid as you put in. With dried material, especially roots, you get out as much as you can. Plants, as they dry, lose their natural moisture content. There are charts available that show how much moisture content many medicinal plants contain. Some plants, such as myrrh gum, contain virtually none, and others, such as mint, contain a great deal.

When making a tincture of a dried plant, you must add back the amount of water that was present in the plant when it was fresh. Generally, dried plants are tinctured at a 5 to 1 ratio (that is, 5 parts liquid to 1 part dried herb). For example, echinacea root contains 30 percent water by weight. If you have 10 ounces powdered echinacea root, you would add to it 50 ounces of liquid (1:5), of

## Combination Tincture Formula for the Liver

*This is a wonderful liver combination made from fresh herbs.*

60 mL (2 ounces) each fresh burdock and
dandelion root tinctures

**To make:** Combine the two tinctures in a 4-ounce (120 mL) amber bottle.
**To use:** For chronic hepatitis, take ½ teaspoon 3 times a day for up to 1 year.

which 35 ounces is 95 percent alcohol and 15 ounces is water. Again, you do not want to use tap water.

To prepare dried herbs for a tincture, powder as fine as possible in a blender or Vita-mix. It is best to store herbs as whole as possible until needed. As with fresh plant tinctures, let the herb–alcohol mixture sit for 2 weeks and then decant.

### Whole Herbs as Powders or in Capsules

Capsules are good for getting a large quantity of herb in whole form into the body. Capsules come in a number of sizes. The most common are "0," "00," and "000," from largest to smallest. The standard size, and that recommended in this book, is "00." Empty capsules are available from most herb stores or mail-order companies (see Resources). They are usually composed of gelatin. I recommend vegetable over animal gelatin for the same reasons I eschew commercial meat.

The herb must be powdered as finely as possible and then encapsulated, a tedious process. I usually try to bribe my son to do it or just buy it ready-made from a retail source. One thing that facilitates encapsulation of herbs is a capsule "machine." It's not really a machine but will make 24 capsules at a time. It is fairly fast and easy: I can make about 125 capsules in 30 minutes.

Sometimes, it is desirable to use powdered herbs in a noncapsule form. For instance, for stomach ulceration, the herbs should be powdered and mixed with liquid and consumed. This allows the herb to make contact with the entire affected area. If the ulceration is in the duodenum, which lies just below the stomach, then capsules would be used. The capsules tend to sit at the bottom of the stomach and then drop through into the duodenum where they are needed. Duodenal ulcers are often accompanied by painful cramps or spasms. This can be alleviated by adding a few drops of peppermint essential oil to the herbal mixture before encapsulating it.

---

## CONSUMING WHOLE HERBS

Many herbs can be harvested and eaten in whole form when needed. Osha root *(Ligusticum porterii)* is a prime example. This herb can be used for sore throats and upper respiratory tract infections of both viral and bacterial origin. It is very strong, and a bit of fresh or dried root can be carried in the pocket and a little of it can be eaten whenever needed. Sometimes, a combination of whole herbs and tinctured herbs works well. For chronic viral hepatitis, a mixture of powdered herbs and a few tinctured herbs seems to work best.

---

I find that loose powered herbs are also good for hepatitis and liver disease. When a large quantity of powdered herb is mixed in juice and consumed before bed, the herbs go into the system quickly and can be processed by the liver extremely rapidly. Because of the large quantities of herbs needed for treatment of hepatitis C, this is the primary means of getting them down easily.

### Children's Dosages

Children are much smaller and are generally more sensitive to herbs than adults. Dosages should be adjusted in herbal medicines for children by using one of these three common approaches.

**Clark's Rule:** Divide the child's weight in pounds by 150 to give an approximate fraction of an adult's dose. For a 75-pound child, the dose would be 75 divided by 150, or half the adult dose.

**Cowling's Rule:** Divide the age of a child at his or her next birthday by 24. For a child who will be 8 years of age, the dose would be 8 divided by 24, or one-third the adult dose.

**Young's Rule:** Divide the child's age by (12 + age of child). For a 3-year-old, the formula is 3 divided by (12 + 3), or 15, for a dose that is one-fifth the adult dose.

### Herbal Glycerites and Honeys

Glycerites and honeys are excellent for children because of their wonderful taste. Additionally, honey as an herbal medium adds its own powerful actions to that of the herb. When making glycerites, use only food-grade vegetable glycerin or organic wildflower honey.

**For dried herbs.** Use 1 part herb to 5 parts liquid, with the liquid composed of 10 percent 95 percent alcohol, 60 percent glycerin or honey, and 30 percent water. If you have 5 ounces of well-powdered echinacea root or goldenseal, you would want 25 ounces of liquid, of which 2.5 ounces would be 95 percent alcohol,

15 ounces would be glycerin or honey, and 7.5 ounces would be water. Mix all liquids well, add powdered dry herb, and leave in a capped Mason jar for 2 weeks; shake the jar daily. Decant and squeeze herb through cloth to extract as much liquid as possible. Store the glycerite or honey in an amber bottle out of the sun.

**For fresh herbs.** Use 1 part herb to 2 parts liquid, composed of 15 percent 95 percent alcohol and 85 percent glycerin or honey. If you have 5 ounces of fresh herb, you would want 10 ounces of liquid, of which 1.5 ounces would be 95 percent alcohol and 8.5 ounces would be glycerin or honey.

**Dosage.** Generally, glycerites and honeys are not as strong as tinctures and may be given at 1½ times the dosage as tinctures. If you would normally give ½ dropper (15 drops) of tincture, you could give ¾ (22 drops) of glycerite or honey.

> ## CAUTION!
>
> As with all medicines, it is important in both adults and children to pay close attention to how the individual is responding to the herbs. Start with small doses and increase gradually. At any sign of adverse reactions, discontinue use of the herb. If severe symptoms persist, consult a competent health care provider.

# RESOURCES

*RECOMMENDED SUPPLIERS FOR HERBS AND MIXTURES*

**Dry Creek Herb Farm**
14245 Edgehill Lane
Auburn, CA 95603
530-888-0889
www.drycreekherbfarm.com
*A source for most of the herbs in this book as well as special formulas for hepatitis, including the formula described in the protocol section and the traditional Chinese formula for minor bupleurum combination. Although this source sometimes has difficulty in obtaining some of the phyllanthus species, it is the only source I know of for bulk phyllanthus and picrorhiza.*

**Dandelion Botanical Company**
708 N. 34th Street
Seattle, WA 98103
206-545-8892
*Has many of the herbs listed in this book.*

**Horizon Seeds**
P.O. Box 69
Williams, OR 97544
541-846-6704
*A source of seeds for many herbs, including several of the Ayurvedic herbs.*

**Hardbody Nutrition**
800-378-6787
www.hardbodynutrition.com
*Carries nutritional supplements and herbs at reasonable prices. Will beat any price by 5 percent. Generally has picroliv, phyllanthol, and n-acetyl-cysteine in stock. Also, search the Web for other sources of these supplements; just type in picroliv or phyllanthol.*

**Wholesale Nutrition**
P.O. Box 3345
Saratoga, CA 95070
800-325-2664
*A source of nutritional supplements, except NAC.*

### HERBAL PRACTITIONERS EXPERIENCED IN THE TREATMENT OF HEPATITIS C

Many clinicians are producing excellent results in the treatment of hepatitis through approaches similar to those described in this book. If you desire a personal health professional, wish a protocol designed especially for you, or have a particularly unique or dangerous manifestation of hepatitis, you may wish to seek out some of these people, all have extensive clinical experience.

**Arizona**
Jesse Stoff, MD
2661 N. Camino De Oeste
Tucson, AZ 84745
602-323-2244
*Conventional physician specializing in chronic fatigue syndrome.*

**California**
Lois Johnson, MD
100 Pleasant Hill Avenue North
Sebastopol, CA 95472
707-829-8750
*Conventional physician highly trained in herbal medicine.*

**Minnesota**
Matthew Wood
6001 Sunnyfield Road
Minnetrista, MN 55364
612-472-8057
*One of the best clinicians in the United States. Heavily trained in homeopathy and western botanic medicine.*

**New York**
Quing Chai Zhang
420 Lexington Avenue
New York, NY 10170
212-573-9584
*TCM practitioner, extensive clinical experience in hepatitis C.*

**Oregon**
Donald Yance
P.O. Box 576
Ashland, OR 97520
541-488-3133
*Specializing in the treatment of cancer; one of the best herbal clinicians in the United States.*

**Washington**
K.P. Khalsa
125 NW 84th Street
Seattle, WA 98117
206-364-2481
*Ayurvedic physician. Exceptionally deep clinical practice for AIDS and other immune disorders.*

**England**
John Tindall
East West Herbs
3 Neals Yard
Covent Garden
London, WC2H 9DP, United Kingdom
44 (0) 171 379 1312
*Specializes in TCM treatment of hepatitis C.*

# SUGGESTED READING

Dolan, Matthew. *The Hepatitis C Handbook.* Berkeley, CA: North Atlantic Books, 1999.

Green, James. *The Herbal Medicine Maker's Handbook.* Forestville, CA: Wildlife and Green Publications, 1990.

Hobbs, Christopher. *Milk Thistle: The Liver Herb.* Loveland, CO: Interweave Press, 1998.

Hobbs, Christopher. *Natural Liver Therapy.* Capitola, CA: Botanica Press, 1997.

Hoffmann, David. *The New Holistic Herbal.* Rockport, MA: Element, 1992.

Landis, R., and K.P. Khalsa. *Herbal Defense.* New York: Warner, 1997.

Margulis, Lynn. *Symbiotic Planet: A New Look at Evolution.* New York: Basic Books, 1998.

Stoff, J., and Charles Pellegrino. *Chronic Fatigue Syndrome: The Hidden Epidemic.* New York: HarperCollins, 1992.

Ryan, Frank. *Virus X: Tracking the New Killer Plagues.* New York: Little, Brown, 1997.

# GLOSSARY

**Acute.** An illness that comes on quickly, has severe symptoms, and, in general, has a short duration (e.g., measles or colds). The opposite of chronic.

**Allopathic.** Conventional modern medicine. Originally, only one of eight or so schools of medicine in the United States were allopathic. By 1930, through a brilliant blend of legislative action, money generation through advertising in *Journal of the American Medical Association,* control over the licensing of medical schools, and deceptive conciliation of other medical organizations, the allopaths gained complete control over American medicine. Prices and quality of health care suffered accordingly.

**Alterative.** A plant or procedure that stimulates physical changes in the body that will appropriately deal with chronic or acute diseases; a substance that renews tissues and improves function slowly and efficiently, culminating in health. Many herbs will show their alterative aspect only in the presence of disease symptoms. In a healthy person, nothing or something entirely different happens. This term is not used in allopathic (conventional) medicine.

**Analgesic.** A substance that relieves pain without unconsciousness.

**Anesthetic.** A substance that decreases the capacity of nerves to experience pain.

**Anodyne.** A substance that eases pain.

**Antibiotic.** A substance that selectively depresses or destroys bacteria (literally, "anti-life").

**Antibody.** An entity in the cells and blood that actively attacks and destroys disease pathogens.

**Anticoagulant.** A substance that slows or stops the clotting of blood.

**Antidepressant.** A substance that counters depression or sadness.

**Antifungal.** A substance that kills or inhibits fungus.

**Antihemorrhagic.** A hemostatic.

**Antihepatotoxic.** A substance that prevents toxins from negatively affecting the liver.

**Antihypertensive.** A substance that lowers blood pressure.

**Anti-inflammatory.** A substance that reduces inflammation.

**Antimicrobial.** A substance that inhibits or kills microorganisms.

**Antimutagenic.** A substance that reduces or interferes with mutagenic activity (that is, the ability to cause mutations) of other substances.

**Antioxidant.** A substance that slows or stops oxidation. In herbalism, specifically one that slows the formation of free radicals.

**Antipyretic.** A substance that reduces fever.

**Antirheumatic.** A substance that eases, prevents, or reduces rheumatic symptoms.

**Antiscorbutic.** A substance that prevents scurvy, usually one that contains vitamin C.

**Antiseptic.** A substance that prevents putrefaction, the decay of cells, and infection.

**Antispasmodic.** A substance that relieves or prevents muscle spasms.

**Antiviral.** A substance that kills viruses or inhibits their reproduction.

**Aperient.** A substance that exerts a mild laxative activity.

**Arteriosclerosis.** A condition in which blood vessels have thickened, hardened, and lost their elasticity because of age or the buildup of fatty plaques along the vessel walls.

**Arthritis.** Inflammation of the joints. Two types: 1) osteoarthritis, a degenerative bone disease involving loss and calcification of joint cartilage (the bones formerly cushioned by gristle now grind together, hurt, and get inflamed), and 2) rheumatoid arthritis, a chronic and increasingly worsening inflammation of the joints from an unknown cause (this type is speculated to be autoimmune, but no one really knows).

**Astringent.** A substance that causes constriction of tissues. In herbal medicine, usually a plant that contains tannins, stops bleeding, and reduces inflammation. In any event, it dries out your mouth if you taste it.

**Bitter tonic.** A bitter-tasting substance that increases gastric secretions, tonifies the stomach, increases deficient appetite, and increases stomach acidity. These substances aid deficient digestion.

**Bronchitis.** Inflammation of bronchial mucous membranes.

**Cardiotonic.** A substance that regulates or strengthens heart action and metabolism; whatever the condition of the heart, a cardiotonic brings it back to within a normal range of action.

**Carminative.** An agent that aids the elimination of gas.

**Cathartic.** A substance that eases griping, expels gas.

**Cholagogue.** A substance that induces gallbladder contraction.

**Choleretic.** A substance that encourages the liver to produce bile.

**Chronic.** A disease of long, slow duration marked by general debility with interspersed acute episodes. The opposite of acute.

**Colitis.** Inflammation of the colon.

**Conjunctivitis.** Inflammation of the mucous membranes of the eye or eyelid.

**Counterirritant.** A substance applied to the skin that produces an irritation, heating, or vasodilating action. It generally speeds healing by increasing blood circulation and warming deep (usually joint) inflammations.

**Demulcent.** A substance that reduces, relieves, or soothes irritation, particularly of mucous membrane surfaces.

**Depurant.** A substance that stimulates excretion.

**Diaphoretic.** A substance that increases perspiration.

**Diuretic.** A substance that increases the flow of urine.

**Duodenum.** The beginning of the small intestine; it lies just beneath the stomach.

**Dysmenorrhea.** Painful menstruation.

**Dyspepsia.** Poor digestion, often with heartburn and stomach acid reflux.

**Eczema.** A chronic allergic skin condition.

**Expectorant.** A substance that causes mucus in the lungs and bronchial tract to come out more easily, usually through coughing.

**Febrifuge.** A substance that reduces fever.

**Gastritis.** Inflammation of the stomach lining.

**Hemostatic.** A substance that slows or stops bleeding.

**Hepatic.** A substance that acts on the liver.

**Hepatitis.** Inflammation of the liver.

**Herb.** A plant used for medicinal or culinary purposes.

**Hypnotic.** An herb that induces sleep.

**Hypotensive.** A substance that lowers blood pressure.

**Immunostimulant.** Something that stimulates the immune system's health and ability to respond to disease, either gradually or quickly.

**Infusion.** An extremely strong tea made with hot or cold water and an herb.

**In vitro.** In a test tube.

**In vivo.** In a live animal.

**Narcotic.** A substance that lessens pain by depressing the central nervous system. Derives from the Greek *narkotikos,* meaning "benumbing."

**Nervine.** A substance that is therapeutic or sedative to the nervous system.

**Neuralgia.** Pain in and originating along nerve fibers.

**Nutritive.** A substance that is ingested and provides nutrition.

**Plant.** Any flora of Earth.

**Pruritis.** Itching. An inflammation of the skin that produces itching.

**Purgative.** A substance that cleanses the bowels.

**Reflux.** The involuntary regurgitation of stomach fluids.

**Refrigerant.** Antipyretic.

**Rhinitis.** Inflammation of the sinus membranes beginning in the mucous membranes of the nose (*rhino* means "nose").

**Sedative.** A substance that has a calming and quieting action on specific organs or systems (cardiac, nervous, cerebral, spinal, respiratory, etc.).

**Soporific.** A substance that produces sleep.

**Spasmolytic.** An antispasmodic substance.

**Stimulant.** A substance that increases the action of a specific organ system or induces a sense and feeling of well-being.

**Sudorific.** A substance that produces sweat.

**Tannins.** Astringent compounds in plants that protect the plant from yeasts, being eaten, and bacterial decay.

**Tincture.** Usually a combination of an herb, alcohol, and water. Created as a result of the preservative and extractive properties of alcohol on herbs.

**Tonic.** A substance taken to strengthen the body or a particular system of the body, generally in the treatment of chronic disease. Loosely, a tonic "tones" whatever system it affects.

**Vulnerary.** A substance used for the healing or treatment of wounds.

**Weed.** A derogatory term for a plant, similar to a racial epithet.

# SELECTED BIBLIOGRAPHY

*Botanical and Supplement References, Primary Sources*

The following books and tapes were primary sources for the herbs, nutritional supplements, foods, and clinical protocols for hepatitis C explored in this book. Journal citations and other specific texts are listed under individual headings. (All audio tapes, except where noted, can be ordered from Tree Farm Communications, 800-468-0464.)

Bergner, Paul. *The Healing Power of Ginseng and the Tonic Herbs.* Rocklin, CA: Prima Publishing, 1996.

Blumenthal, Mark, et al. *The Complete German Commission E Monographs.* Austin, TX: American Botanical Council, 1998.

Cech, Richo. *Horizon Herbs: Growing Guide and Catalog Preview 2000.* Williams, OR: Horizon Seeds, 1999.

Dolan, Matthew. *The Hepatitis C Handbook.* Berkeley, CA: North Atlantic Books, 1999.

Duke, James. *The Green Pharmacy.* Emmaus, PA: Rodale Press, 1998.

Ellingwood, Finley. *American Materia Medica, Therapeutics, and Pharmacognosy.* Cincinnati, OH: Eclectic Publications, 1919.

Felter, H., and John Uri Lloyd. *King's American Dispensatory.* Cincinnati, OH: Eclectic Publications, 1895.

Foster, S., and Yue Chongxi. *Herbal Emissaries.* Rochester, VT: Healing Arts Press, 1992.

Fulder, Stephen. *The Book of Ginseng (and Other Chinese Herbs for Vitality).* Rochester, VT: Healing Arts Press, 1993.

Hobbs, Christopher. *Natural Liver Therapy.* Capitola, CA: Botanica Press, 1997.

Hoffmann, David. *The New Holistic Herbal.* Rockport, MA: Element, 1992.

Landis, R., and K.P. Khalsa. *Herbal Defense.* New York: Warner, 1997.

Leung, Alfred. *Chinese Herbal Remedies.* New York: Universe Books, 1984.

Majupuria, Trilock. *Religious and Useful Plants of Nepal and India.* Lashkar, India: Craftsman Press, 1989.

Moerman, Daniel. *Medicinal Plants of Native America.* Ann Arbor, MI: University of Michigan, Museum of Anthropology, Technical reports, Number 19, 1986.

Moore, Michael. *Herbal Materia Medica.* Albuquerque, NM: Southwest School of Botanical Medicine, 1994.

———. *Medicinal Plants of the Pacific West.* Sante Fe, NM: Red Crane Books, 1993.

———. *Medicinal Plants of the Mountain West.* Sante Fe, NM: Museum of New Mexico Press, 1979.

Mowrey, Daniel. *The Scientific Validation of Herbal Medicine.* New Canaan, CT: Keats, 1986. Multiple studies are cited in this book.

Nadkarni, K.M. *Indian Materia Medica.* Bombay: Popular Prakashan, 1976.

Reid, Daniel. *Chinese Herbal Medicine.* Boston: Shambhala, 1993.

"Therapeutic approaches to viral hepatitis." *Protocol Journal of Botanic Medicine* 1 (1995 2):129–172. Multiple citations are listed.

Weed, Susun S. *Healing Wise.* Woodstock, NY: Ash Tree, 1989.

Weil, Andrew. *Eight Weeks to Optimum Health.* New York: Knopf, 1998.

Weiss, Rudolph. *Herbal Medicine.* Gothenberg, Sweden: Beaconsfield, 1988.

Werbach, M., and Michael Murray. *Botanical Influences on Illness.* Tarzana, CA: Third Line Press, 1994. This book cites numerous research studies.

Wood, Matthew. *The Book of Herbal Wisdom.* Berkeley, CA: North Atlantic Books, 1997.

NAPRALERT database. NAPRALERT is an acronym for Natural Products ALERT, a dynamic database that is updated periodically and has been copyrighted from 1975 to date by the Board of Trustees, The University of Illinois. NAPRALERT is maintained by the Program for Collaborative Research in the Pharmaceutical Sciences, within the Department of Medicinal Chemistry and Pharmacognosy at the College of Pharmacy of the University of Illinois at Chicago, 833 South Wood Street (mailcode 877), Chicago, IL 60612; 312-996-2246. The data in NAPRALERT represent a synthesis of information from more than 150,000 scientific journal articles, books, abstracts, and patents, collected systematically from the global literature since 1975.

### Clinician Tapes

Alschuler, Lise. *Supporting the Liver with Botanicals.* 43rd Annual Northwest Naturopathic Physicians Convention. May 21–23, 1999. Audio tape.

Barrie, Stephen. *The Role of Intestinal and Liver Detoxification Processes in Health and Disease.* Great Smokies Diagnostic Laboratory, tape #4. No date provided.

Bauer, Carl Hangee. *Naturopathic Treatment of Hepatitis C.* 14th Annual American Association of Naturopathic Physicians Convention, November 3–7, 1999. Audio tape.

Cheney, Paul, MD. *Evidence for Glutathione Deficiency in Chronic Fatigue Syndrome.* Conference on Bioenergetic Medicine, February 5–7, 1999. Audio tape.

James, Mary. *Liver Detoxification and the Gut Connection.* Northwest Naturopathic Physicians Convention, 1995. Audio tape.

Myers, Robert. *Understanding Viral Hepatitis.* Arizona Naturopathic Medical Association 1996 Annual Convention, December 6–8, 1996. Audio tape.

O'Connor, Diedre. *Optimizing Liver Function with Botanicals.* Gaia Naturopathic Herb Symposium, 1993. Audio tape.

Phounasavan, Say Fone. *300 Chronic Hepatitis B Patients Treated with Oriental Herbs.* American Association of Naturopatic Physicians, 1987. Audio tape.

Tierra, Michael. *Liver: Comparing Western and Chinese Medicine.* Traditional Healing Conference, 1992. Audio tape.

Tillotson, Alan. *Classic Ayurvedic Treatment for Hepatitis.* 10th Annual American Herbalist Guild Symposium, August 5–8, 1999. Audio tape.

Wilson, Richard. *Viral Hepatitis—Diagnosis and Treatment.* 36th Annual NWNP Convention, May 13–15, 1993. Audio tape.

Yance, Donald. *Hepatitis C: Managing Chronic Hepatitis with Botanical Medicines.* Medicines From the Earth Conference, 1999. Available from Herbal Education Services 800-252-0688.

Yance, D., Lois Johnson, and Michael Moore. Hepatitis Panel. Breitenbush Herb Conference, August 27–29, 1999. Audio tape.

### Journal Citations and Specific Plant References

All journal citations followed by "NC" are NAPRALERT citations. Because of space limitations (and given that I had 50 to 100 citations for most of these herbs), it was possible to include only a representative sampling of the journal citations.

### Emerging Viruses, Coevolution, and Viral Intelligence

Garret, Laurie. *The Coming Plague.* New York: Farrar, Straus, Giroux, 1994.

Margulis, L., and René Fester, editors. *Symbiosis as a Source of Evolutionary Evolution.* Cambridge, MA: MIT Press, 1991.

Margulis, L., and Dorian Sagan. *Microcosmos: Four Billion Years of Microbial Evolution.* New York: Simon & Schuster, 1986.

Margulis, Lynn. *Symbiotic Planet.* New York: Basic Books, 1998.

Peters, C.J. *Virus Hunter.* New York: Doubleday, 1997.

Preston, Richard. "The Demon in the Freezer." *The New Yorker:* 44–60. 12 July 1999.

———. *The Hot Zone.* New York: Random House, 1997.

Roberts, D. McL. et al, editors. *Evolution of Microbial Life.* New York: Cambridge University Press, 1996.

Ryan, Frank. *Virus X: Tracking the New Killer Plagues.* New York: Little, Brown, 1997.

Stoff, J., and Charles Pellegrino. *Chronic Fatigue Syndrome: The Hidden Epidemic.* New York: HarperCollins, 1992.

## Food Herbs, Additional Sources

Bewicke, Dhyana, et al. *Chlorella: The Emerald Food.* Berkeley, CA: Ronin, 1984.

Challem, Jack. *Spirulina.* New Canaan, CT: Keats, 1981.

Elkins, Rita. *Blue-Green Algae.* Pleasant Grove, UT: Woodland, 1995.

Hills, Christopher. *The Secrets of Spirulina.* Boulder Creek, CA: University of the Trees Press, 1980.

Koch, Heinrich, and L. Dawson. *Garlic: The Science and Therapeutic Application of* Allium sativum *and Related Species.* Baltimore, MD: Williams & Wilkins, 1996.

Lee, William, and M. Rosenbaum. *Chlorella.* New Canaan, CT: Keats, 1987.

Rosen, Diana. *The Book of Green Tea.* Pownal, VT: Storey, 1998.

Switzer, Larry. *Spirulina: The Whole Food Revolution.* Berkeley, CA: Proteus, 1980.

Udall, Kate. *Green Tea.* Pleasant Grove, UT: Woodland, 1998.

NAPRALERT citations as of October 1999 for all food herbs effective in alleviating liver disease.

## Immune Herbs, Additional Sources

### ASHWAGANDHA

Al-hindawi, M.K., et al. "Anti-granuloma activity of Iraqi *Withania somnifera.*" *J Ethnopharmacol* 37 (1992 2):113–116. NC

———. "Anti-inflammatory activity of some Iraqi plants using intact rats." *J Ethnopharmacol* 26 (1989 2):163–168. NC

Anabalagan, K., et al. "*Withania somnifera* (ashwagandha), a rejuvinating herbal drug which controls alpha-2-macroglobulin synthesis during inflammation." *Int J Crude Drug Res* 23 (1985 4):177–183. NC

Babbar, O.P., et al. "Evaluation of plants for antiviral activity." *Indian J Med Res Suppl* 76 (1982):54–65. NC

Bhargava, K.P., et al. "Antistress activity in Indian medicinal plants." *J Res Edu Indian Med* 4 (1985 3/4):27–31. NC

Bhattacharya, S.K., et al. "Antioxidant activity of glycowithanolides from *Withania somnifera.*" *Indian J Exp Biol* 35 (1997 3): 236–239. NC

Chhajed, S., et al. "Evaluation of hepato-protective effect of *Piper longum* and *Withania somnifera* in hepatotoxicity induced by antitubercular drugs in mice." *J Res Edu Indian Med* 10 (1991 3): 9–12. NC

Dhuley, J.N. "Therapeutic efficacy of ashwagandha against experimental aspergillosis in mice." *Immunopharmacol Immunotoxicol* 20 (1998 1):191–198. NC

Gupta, O.P., et al. "Pharmacological investigations of *Withania somnifera* (ashwagandha) as an adaptogen." *Indian J Pharmacy* 39 (1977):163A. NC

Hattori, M., et al. "Inhibitory effects of various Ayurvedic and Panamanian medicinal plants on the infection of herpes simplex virus-1 in vitro and in vivo." *Phytother Res* 9 (1995 4):270–276. NC

Hirobe, C., et al. "Screening test for antitumor activity of crude drugs (IV). Studies on cytotoxic activity of Israeli medicinal plants." *Nat Med* 48 (1994 2):168–170. NC

Kulkarni, R.R., et al. "Treatment of osteoarthritis with a herbomineral formulation: a double-blind, placebo-controlled, cross-over study." *J Ethnopharmacol* 33 (1991 1/2):91–95. NC

Mehta, A.K., et al. "Pharmacological effects of *Withania somnifera* root extract of GABA receptor complex." *Indian J Med Res* 94 (1991 4):312–315. NC

Montilla, M.P., et al. "The protective and curative action of *Withania frutescens* leaf extract against $CCl_4$-induced hepatotoxicity." *Phytother Res* 4 (1990 6):212–215. NC

Panda, S., et al. "Protective role of ashwagandha in cadmium-induced hepatotoxicity and nephrotoxicity in male mouse." *Curr Sci* 72 (1997 8):546–547. NC

Singh, N., et al. "Indian plants as anti-stress agents." Abstr International Res Con Nat Prod Coll Pharm Univ N Carolina, July 7–12, 1985. NC

Singh, N., et al. "*Withania somnifera* (ashwagandha), a rejuvinating herbal drug which enhances survival during stress (an adaptogen)." *Int J Crude Drug Res* 20 (1982 1):29–35. NC

Sudhir, S., et al. "Pharmacological studies on leaves of *Withania somnifera*." *Planta Med* 52 (1986 1):61–63. NC

ASTRAGALUS

Cao, G.W., et al. "Influence of four kinds of polysaccharides on the induction of lymphokine-activated killer cells in vivo." *J Med Coll Pla* 8 (1993 1):5–11. NC

Chang, C.Y., et al. "Effect of *Astragalus membranaceus* on enhancement of mouse killer cell activity." *Chung-kuo I Hseuh K'o Hseuh Yuan Hseuh Pao* 5 (1983 4):231–234. NC

Chu, D.T., et al. "Immunotherapy with Chinese medicinal herbs I. Immune restoration of local xenogeneic graft-vs-host reaction in cancer patients by fractionated *Astragalus membranaceus* in vitro." *J Clin Lab Immunol* 25 (1988 3):119–123. NC

Chu, D.T., et al. "Immunotherapy with Chinese medicinal herbs II. Reversal of cyclophosphamide-induced immune suppression by administration of fractionated *Astragalus membranaceus* in vivo." *J Clin Lab Immunol* 25 (1988 3):125–129. NC

Hou, Y., et al. "Effect of *Radix astragali sur hedysari* on the interferon system." *Chinese Med J* 94 (1981 1):35–40. NC

"Immunity parameters and blood cAMP changes in normal persons after ingestion of *Radix astragali*." *Natl Med J China* 59 (1979):31–34. NC

Jin, R., et al. "Immunomodulative effects of Chinese herbs in mice treated with anti-tumor agent cyclophosphamide." *Yakugaku Zasshi* 114 (1994 7):533–538. NC

Kajimura, K., et al. "Pharmacological quality of *Astragali radix*; the effect of antibody production in vitro." *Nat Med* 51 (1997 1):45–49. NC

Kumazawa N., et al. "Protective effects of various methanol extracts of crude drugs on experimental hepatic injury induced by alpha-naphthylisothiocyanate in rats." *Yakugaku Zasshi* 111 (1991 3):199–204. NC

Lau, B.H.S., et al. "Macrophage chemiluminescence modulated by Chinese medicinal herbs *Astragalus membranaceus, Ligustrum lucidum*." *Phytother Res* 3 (1989 4):148–153. NC

Lee, J.H. "Antineoplastic natural products and the analogues. XI. Cytotoxic activity against L1210 cell of some raw drugs from oriental medicine and folklore." *Korean J Pharmacog* 17 (1986 4):286–291. NC

Lee, J.W., et al. "Screening of medicinal plants having hepatoprotective activity effect with primary cultured hepatocytes intoxicated with carbon tetrachloride cytotoxicity." *Korean J Pharmacog* 23 (1992 4):268–275. NC

Li, Y.Y., et al. "Induction characteristic of lymphoblastoid interferon." *Chung-kuo I Hseuh K'o Hseuh Yuan Hseuh Pao* 2 (1980):250–253. NC

Ma, R., et al. "The effect of *Radix astragali* on mouse marrow hemopoieses." *J Trad Chinese Med* 3 (1983 3):199–204. NC

McCaleb, Rob. "Astragalus for the liver." *HerbalGram* 25 (summer 1991):19, citing Yang, Y.Z., et al., *Chinese Med J* 107 (1987 7):595.

———. "Astragalus enhances natural killer cell activity." *HerbalGram* 21 (fall 1989):16, citing *J Clin Lab Immunol* 25 (1988):112–123.

———. "Immune system stimulation from astragalus." *HerbalGram* 17 (summer 1988):24, citing *Cancer Research,* 48 (1988):1410–1415.

Qian, Z.W., et al. "Synergism of *Astragalus membranaceus* with interferon in the treatment of cervical erosion and their antiviral activities." *Chung Hsi I Chieh Ho Tsa Chih* 7 (1987 5):268–269. NC

Shirataki, Y., et al. "Antioxidative components isolated from the roots of *Astragalus membranaceus bunge (Astragali radix)." *Phytother Res* 11 (1997 8):603–605. NC

Sun, Y., et al. "Immune restoration and/or augmentation of local graft versus host reaction by traditional Chinese medicinal herbs." *Cancer* 52 (1983):70–73. NC

Wang, D.C., et al. "Influence of *Astragalus membranaceus* (Am) polysaccharide FB on immunologic function of human periphery blood lymphocyte." *Chung-hua Chung Liu Tsa Chih* 11 (1989 3):180–183. NC

Wang, W.Y,. et al. "Effect of *Astragalus membranaceus* on the cytokine production in aged subjects." *Zhongguo Mianyixue Zazhi* 11 (1995 3):167–169. NC

Yang, Y.Z., et al. "Effect of *Astragalus membranaceus* on natural killer cell activity and induction of alpha- and gamma-interferon in patients with coxsackie B viral myocarditis." *Chung-hus I Hseuh Chih (English Edition)* 103 (1990 4):304–307. NC

Yoshida, Y., et al. "Immunomodulating activity of Chinese herbs and *Oldenlandia diffusa* in particular." *Int J Immuno-pharmacol* 39 (1997 7):359–370. NC

Zhang, Y.D., et al. "Effects of astragalus (ASI, SK) on experimental liver injury." *Yao Hseuh Hseuh Pao* 27 (1992 6):401–406. NC

Zhang, Z.L., et al. "Hepatoprotective effects of astragalus root." *J Ethnopharmacol* 30 (1990 1):91–95. NC

Zhuang, M.X., et al. "Effects of some medicinal polysaccharides on immune deficiency in animal models induced by cobra anticomplementary factor." *J Nat Toxins* 5 (1996 2):161–164. NC

Zuang, M.X. "The effects of polysaccharides of *Astragalus membranaceus, Codonopsis pilosula, Panax ginseng* on some immune functions in guinea pigs." *Zhonghua Yaoxue Zazhi* 27 (1988 11):653–655. NC

Zuo, L., et al. "The curative effects of *Astragalus membranaceus* bungo A6 fraction in combination with acyclovir on mice infected with HSV-1." *Zhongguo Bingduxue* 10 (1995 2):177–179. NC

## BONESET

Bergner, Paul. *The Healing Power of Echinacea and Goldenseal.* Rocklin, CA: Prima Publishing, 1997.

Boyd, L. "Pharmacology of the homeopathic drugs." *J Am Inst Homeopathy* 21 (1928):209. NC

Gassinger, C., et al. "A controlled clinical trial for testing the efficacy of the homeopathic drug *Eupatorium perfoliatum* D2 in the treatment of common cold." *Arzneimittelforschung* 31 (1981):732–736. NC

Muni, I., et al. "Cytotoxicity of North Dakota plants I: in vitro studies." *J Pharm Sci* 56 (1967):50–54. NC

Vollmar, A., et al. "Immunologically active polysaccharides of *Eupatorium cannabinum* and *Eupatorium perfoliatum.*" *Phytochemistry* 25 (1986 2):377–381. NC

Wagner, H., et al. Immunostimulating polysaccharides of higher plants." *Arzneimittelforschung* 35 (1985 7):1069–1075. NC

Wagner, H., et al. Immunostimulating polysaccharides of higher plants/preliminary communication." *Arzneimittelforschung* 34 (1984 6):659–661. NC

## CODONOPSIS

Chang, I.M., et al. "Screening of Korean medicinal plants for antitumor activity." *Arch Pharm Res* 3 (1980 2):75–78. NC

Choi, S.Y., et al. "Plants with liver protective activities." *Ann Rep Nat Prod Res Inst Seoul Natl Univ* 21 (1982):49–53. NC

Ch'u, L.H. "The use of 'wen-pu Chu-shui Huan' to treat ascites of late stage schistosomiasis." *Chiang-su Chung-I* 7 (1965):38–39. NC

Han, B.H., et al. "Screening on the anti-inflammatory activity of crude drugs." *Korean J Pharmacog* 4 (1972 3):205–209. NC

Kim, Y.S., et al. "Effects of traditional drugs on $CCl_4$-induced cytotoxicity in primary cultured rat hepatocytes." *Korean J Pharmacog* 25 (1994 4):388–394. NC

Lee, I.R., et al. "A study on the physiological activity of *Codonopsis ussuriensis.*" *Korean J Pharmacog* 20 (1989 4):233–242. NC

Liu, G. "Recent studies on the chemical constituents and pharmacological actions of dangshen *(Codonopsis pilosula).*" *Chin J Integ Trad West Med* 3 (1983 2):114–117. NC

Mseng, Y.S., et al. "Antioxidant activity of ethanol extract from dodok *(Codonopsis lanceolata)." Han'guk Sinp'um Kwahakoe Chi* 23 (1991 3):311–316. NC

Zhuang, M.X., et al. "Effects of some medicinal polysaccharides on immune deficiency in animal models induced by cobra anticomplementary factor." *J Nat Toxins* 5 (1996 2):161–164. NC

Zuang, M.X., "The effects of polysaccharides of *Astragalus membranaceus, Codonopsis pilosula, Panax ginseng* on some immune functions in guinea pigs." *Zhonghua Yaoxue Zazhi* 27 (1988 11):653–655. NC

## LICORICE

Acharya, S., et al. "A preliminary open trial on interferon stimulator derived from *Glycyrrhiza glabra* in the treatment of subacute hepatic failure." *Indian J Med Res* 98 (1993 2):69–74. NC

Bannister, B. "Cardiac arrest due to liquorice-induced hypokalemia." *Br Med J* 2 (1977):738. NC

Chang, I.M., et al. "Plants with liver protective activities." In: *Advances in Chinese Medicinal Materials Research.* H.M. Chang, et al., editors. Philadelphia: World Press, 1984:269–285. NC

Goto, W., et al. "Suppression of hepatitis B surface antigen secretion by traditional plant medicines." *Phytother Res* 10 (1996 6):504–507. NC

Hrelia, P., et al. "Potential antimutagenic activity of *Glycyrrhiza glabra* extract." *Phytother Res* 10 (1996):S101–S103. NC

Kumazawa, N., et al. "Protective effects of various methanol extracts of crude drugs on experimental hepatic injury induced by carbon tetrachloride in rats." *Yakugaku Zashi* 110 (1990 12):950–957. NC

Ngo, H., et al. "Modulation of mutagenesis, DNA binding, and metabolism of aflatoxin B1 by licorice compounds." *Nutr Res* 12 (1992 2):247–257. NC

Okada, K., et al. "Identification of antimicrobial and antioxidant constituents from licorice of Russian and Xinjiang origin." *Chem Pharm Bull* 37 (1989 9):2528–2530. NC

Park, E.J., et al. "Antifibrotic effects of a polysaccharide extracted from *Ganoderma lucidum, glycyrrhizin,* and pentoxifylline in rats with cirrhosis induced by biliary obstruction. *Biol Pharm Bull* 20 (1997 4):417–420. NC

Shirinyan, E., et al. "9,11,13-trihydroxy-10(e)-ocadecenic and 9,12,13-trihydroxy-10,11-epoxoctadecaonic acids. New antistressor compounds from liquorice. *IZV Akad Nauk SSR* 6 (1988):932–936. NC

Sigurjonsdottir, H., et al. "Is blood pressure commonly raised by moderate consumption of liquorice?" *J Human Hypertens* 9 (1995 5):345–348. NC

Sitohy, M.Z., et al. "Metabolite effects of licorice roots *(Glychrrhiza glabra)* on lipid distribution pattern, liver and renal function of albino rats." *Nahrung* 35 (1991 8):799–806. NC

Snow, Joanne. "*Glycyrrhiza glabra.*" *Protocol Journal of Botanical Medicine* 1 (winter 1996 3):9–14.

Taylor, A., and F. Bartter. "Hypertension in licorice intoxication, acromegaly, and Cushing's syndrome." *Hypertens Physiopathol Treat* 755(1977). NC

Wang G.S., and Z.W. Han. "Effects of flavonoids of glycyrrhiza on ethanol-induced liver injury in mice." *Zhongguo Yaolixue Tongbao* 9 (1993 4):271–273. NC

Wang, G.S., and Z.W. Han. "The protective action of glycyrrhiza flavonoids against carbon tetrachloride hepatotoxicity in mice" *Yao Hseuh Hseuh Pao* 28 (1993 8):572–576. NC

Watanabe, S., et al. "Release of secretin of liquorice extract in dogs." *Pancreas* 1 (1986 5):449–454. NC

Yun, H.S., et al. "Liver protective activities of Korean medicinal plants." *Korean J Pharmacog* 11 (1980):149–152. NC

## PANAX GINSENG

Davydov, V.V., et al. "Efficacy of ginseng drugs in experimental insulin-dependent diabetes and toxic hepatitis." *Patol Fiziol Ekspter* 5 (1990):49–52. NC

Goto, W., et al. "Suppression of hepatitis B surface antigen secretion by traditional plant medicines." *Phytother Res* 10 (1996 6):504–507. NC

Han, B.K., et al. "Studies on the effectiveness of ginseng preparations." *Korean J Pharmacog* 15 (1984 2):98–103. NC

Hikino, H. "Antihepatotoxic activity of crude drugs." *Yakugaku Zasshi* 105 (1985 2):109–118. NC

Jeong, T.C., et al. "Protective effects of red ginseng saponins against carbon tetrachloride-induced hepatotoxicity in Sprague Dawley rats." *Planta Med* 63 (1997 2):136–140. NC

Joo, CN. "Some biochemical effects of saponin fraction of *Panax ginseng.*" *Korean J Ginseng Sci* 16 (1992 1):53–63. NC

Kim S.Y., et al. "The effect of ginsenosides on galactosamine-induced hepatotoxicity." *Korean J Pharmacog* 22 (1991 4):219–224. NC

———. "Protective effect of ginseng polysaccharide fraction on $CCl_4$-induced hepatotoxicity in vitro and in vivo." *Koryo Insam Hakhoechi* 19 (1995 2):108–113. NC

Ko, K.M., et al. "Study on animal liver excretion function affected by administration of Korean ginseng glycoside." *Yakhak Hoe Chi* 20 (1976):119. NC

Lin, J.H., et al. "Effects of ginseng on the blood chemistry profile of dexamethasone-treated male rats." *Am J Chinese Med* 23 (1995 2):167–172. NC

Park, J.D., et al. "A comparative biological study of the rhizome and main root from red and white ginsengs." *Korean J Ginseng Sci* 20 (1996 3):256–261. NC

Song, J.H., et al. "Effects of Panax ginseng on galactosamine-induced cytotoxicity in primary cultured rat hepatocytes." *Yakhak Hoe Chi* 34 (1990 5):341–347. NC

Wang, B.X., et al. "The effect of saponin isolated from stems and leaves of ginseng on experimental liver injury." *Yao Hsueh Hsueh Pao* 22 (1987 9):650–654. NC

Yu, H.Y., et al. "An experimental study on the effect of ginseng saponin upon alcoholic liver injury." *Hanyang Uidae Haksaulchi* 2 (1982 2):287–304. NC

Zuang, M.X. "The effects of polysaccharides of *Astragalus membranaceus, Codonopsis pilosula, Panax ginseng* on some immune functions in guinea pigs." *Zhonghua Yaoxue Zazhi* 27 (1988 11):653–655. NC

Zuin, M., et al. "Effects of a preparation containing a standardized ginseng extract combined with trace elements and multivitamins against hepato-toxin-induced chronic liver disease in the elderly." *J Int Med Res* 15 (1987 5):276–281. NC

RED ROOT

Groot, J.T. "The pharmacology of *Ceanothus americanus* I. Preliminary studies on hemodynamics and the effects on coagulation." *J Pharmacol Exp Ther* 30 (1927):275–291. NC

Lynch, T.A., and T.S. Miya. "An investigation of the blood coagulating principles from *Ceanothus americanus*." Dissertation abstract, Int B 27:562–, 1966. NC

Nakanishi, T., et al. "Antiviral and antitumor activities of some western North American plants with surface exudates (1). Inhibitory effects on HIV-1 reverse transcriptase." *Shoyakugaku Zasshi* 47 (1993 3):295–300. NC

SCHIZANDRA

Aburada, M., et al. "Pharmaceuticals containing schisandrin derivatives for the treatment of liver failure." Patent. Pct Int Appl Wo-86 07, 256, 1987. NC

Ahumada, F., et al. "Studies on the effect of *Schizandra chinensis* extract on horses submitted to exercise and maximum effort." *Phytother Res* 3 (1989 5):175–179. NC

Amirov, R.O., et al. "The problem of the nonspecific elevation by drugs of the resistance of the body to the action of toxic substances." *Uch Zap Azerb Inst Usoversch Vrachei* 1 (1966):3. NC

"Effects of gossypol on serum transaminases of rats." *Shan-Hsi-Hsin I Yao* 9 (1980 8):46–49. NC

Hancke, J.L., et al. "Antidepressant activity of selected natural products." *Planta Med* 6 (1986):542–543. NC

Hancke, J., et al. "Reduction of serum hepatic transaminases and CPK in sport horses with poor performance treated with a standardized *Schizandra chinensis* fruit extract." *Phytomedicine* 3 (1996 3):237–240. NC

Hendrich, S., et al. "Effects of dietary brussel sprouts, *Illicium verum, Schizandra chinensis* on carcinogen metabolism systems in mouse liver." *Food Chem Toxicol* 24 (1989 9):903–912. NC

———. "Effects of dietary cabbage, brussel sprouts, *Illicium verum, Schizandra chinensis* and alfalfa on the benzopyrene metabolic system in mouse liver." *Food Chem Toxicol* 21 (1983 4):479–486. NC

Hikino, H. "Antihepatotoxic activity of crude drugs." *Yakugaku Zasshi* 105 (1985 2):109–118. NC

Kim, M.S., et al. "Immunopotentiating activity of water extracts of some crude drugs." *Korean J Pharmacog* 19 (1988 3):193–200. NC

Kim, Y.S., and K.H. Park. "Effects of traditional drugs on CCl$_4$-induced cytotoxicity in primary cultured rat hepatocytes." *Korean J Pharmacog* 245 (1994 4):388–394. NC

Ko, K.M., et al. "Protective effect of a lignan-enriched extract of *Fructus schisandrae* on physical exercise induced muscle damage in rats." *Phytother Res* 10 (1996 5):450–452. NC

———. "Enhancement of hepatic glutathione regeneration capacity by a lignan-enriched extract of *Fructus schisandrae* in rats." *Jpn J Pharmacol* 69 (1995 4):439–442. NC

———. "*Schisandra chinensis*-derived antioxidant activities in 'sheng mai san,' a compound formulation, in vivo, in vitro." *Phytother Res* 9 (1995 3):203–206.

Li, M., et al. "Effect of the oil emulsion of *Schisandra chinensis* on the incorporation of thymidine into the DNA of lymphocytes." *Yao Hsueh T'ung Pao* 17 (1982 5):307–. NC

Liu, G.T., et al. "A comparison of the protective actions of biphenyl dimethyl-dicarboxylate trans-stilbene, alcoholic extracts of *Fructus schizandrae* and *Ganoderma lucidum* against experimental liver injury in mice." *Yao Hsueh Hsueh Pao* 14 (1979):598–604. NC

———. "Induction of hepatic microsomal cytochrome P-450 by scizandrin B in mice." Proceedings of the U.S.-China Pharmacology Symposium, October 29–31, 1979. National Academy of Sciences, 1980, 301–313. NC.

Liu, G.T., and H.L. Wei. "Protection by *Fructus schizandrae* against acetaminophen hepatotoxicity in mice." *Yao Hsueh Hsueh Pao* 22 (1987 9):650–654. NC

Nishiyama, N., et al. "Beneficial effects of s-113m, a novel herbal prescription, on learning impairment model in mice." *Biol Pharm Bull* 18 (1995 1):1498–1503. NC

Pao, T.T., et al. "Studies on schizandra fruit. I. Its effect on increased SGPT levels in animals caused by hepatotoxic chemical agents." *Natl Med J China* 54 (1974):275–. NC

Shipochliev, I., et al. "Pharmacologic study of Bulgarian *Schizandra chinensis*." *Farmatsiya (Sofia)* 17 (1967 3):56–. NC.

Thabrew, M.R., and R.D. Hughes. "Phytogenic agents in the therapy of liver disease." *Phytother Res* 10 (1996 6):461–467. NC

Toda, S., et al. "Natural antioxidants (IV). Antioxidative components isolated from schisandra fruit." *Shoyakugaku Zasshi* 42 (1988 2):156–159. NC

## SIBERIAN GINSENG

Foster, Steven. *Siberian Ginseng*. Austin, TX: American Botanical Council; 1991.

Kim, C.J., and D.R. Hahn. "The biological activity of a new glycoside, chiisanoside, from *Acanthopanax chiisanensis* nakai leaves." *Yakhak Hoe Chi* 24 (1980):123–134. NC

Kim, Y.S., and K.H. Park. "Effects of traditional drugs on CCl$_4$-induced cytotoxicity in primary cultured rat hepatocytes." *Korean J Pharmacog* 245 (1994 4):388–394. NC

Li, S.E. "Effect of eleutherococcus glycosides on the mitotic cycle of regenerating liver hepatocytes." *Lek Sredstva Dal'nego Vostoka* 11 (1972):70. NC

McCaleb, Rob. "Nature's Medicine for Memory Loss." *HerbalGram* 23 (summer 1990):15.

Shen, M.L., et al. "Immunopharmacological effects of polysaccharides from *Acanthopanax senticosus* on experimental animals." *Int J Immunopharmacol* 13 (1991 5):549–554. NC

## TIENCHI GINSENG

Chen, Q.H., et al. "Pharmacology of total saponins of the fibrous roots of *Panax notoginseng.*" *Chung Yao T'ung Pao* 12 (1987 3):173–175. NC

Dua, P.R., et al. "Adaptogenic activity of Indian panax pseudoginseng." *Indian J Exp Biol* 27 (1989 7):631–634. NC

Fan, P., and L. Shi. "Main saponins of notoginseng and ginseng ginsenosides decrease the contents of tissue lipofuscin and serum lipid peroxides in old rats." *Zhongguo Yaolixue Yu Dulixue Zazhi* 2 (1988 4):257–260. NC

Gao, H., et al. "Immunostimulating polysaccharides from *Panax notoginseng.*" *Pharmaceut Res* 13 (1996 8):1196–1200. NC

Gong, Z., et al. "Study of superoxide anion-scavenging effect of ginsenoside-related glycosides." *Zhongguo Yaoke Daxue Xuebao* 22 (1991 1):41–43. NC

Goto, W., et al. "Suppression of hepatitis B surface antigen secretion by traditional plant medicines." *Phytother Res* 10 (1996 6):504–507. NC

"Injection made from shensanqi *(Panax pseudo-ginseng)* and its anti-hepatitis effects." *Chung Ts'ao Yao* 12 (1981 3):14–15. NC

Konoshima, T., et al. "Antitumor promoting activities of the roots of *Panax notoginseng.*" *Nat Med* 50 (1996 2):158–162. NC

Lei, M., et al. "Treatment of 80 patients with hyperlipidemia with the Chinese traditional medicine 'yishou.'" *Phytother Res* 4 (1990 4):165–. NC

Li, X.L., et al. "Protective effects of panaztriol saponins (pts) isolated from *Panax notoginseng* on ischemic-reperfused injury and arrhythmia in isolated rat hearts." *Zhongguo Yaoixue Yu Dulixue Zazhi* 6 (1992 4):272–274. NC

Lin, S.G., et al. "Effect of *Panax notoginseng* saponins on increased proliferation of cultured aortic smooth muscle cells stimulated by hypercholesterolemic serum." *Chung-kuo Yao Li Hsueh Pao* 14 (1993 4):314–316. NC

Lin, W.S., et al. "Superoxide and traditional Chinese medicines." *J Ethnopharmacol* 48 (1995 3):165–171. NC

Liu, J., et al. "The effect of Chinese hepato-protective medicines on experimental liver injury in mice." *J Ethnopharmacol* 42 (1994 3):183–191. NC

Ma, L.Y., et al. "Effects of *Panax notoginseng* saponins on platelet aggregation in rats with middle cerebral artery occlusion or in vitro and on lipid fluidity of platelet membrane." *Phytother Res* 12 (1998 2):138–140. NC

Pan, H.P., et al. "Experimental studies on the anti-aging effect of total saponin from stalk and leaf of sanchi *(Panax notoginseng)*." *Chung Ts'ao Yao* 24 (1993 11):581–584. NC

Prasain, J.K., et al. "Hepatoprotective effects of *Panax notoginseng*: ginsenosided -re and -rgi as its active constituents in D-galactosamine/lipopolysaccharide-induced liver injury." *Phytomedicine* 2 (1996 4):297–303. NC

Sasaki, R., et al. "Antitumor polysaccharides from *Panax notoginseng* roots." Patent. Japan Kokai Tokkyo Koho-02 268, 120, 1990. NC

Song, L.C., et al. "Effects of total saponins of *Panax notoginseng* on DNA and protein metabolism in mice intoxicated with $CCl_4$." *Yao Hseuh T'ung Pao* 17 (1982 2):67–69. NC

Xu, Q., et al. "Blood lipid-decreasing action of total saponins of panax notoginseng." *Zhongguo Zhongyao Zazhi* 18 (1993 6):367–368. NC

Zhang, B., et al. "Effects of *Panax notoginseng* (76017) on myocardial ischemia, cyclic nucleotides, nucleic acid and protein." *He Jishu* 2 (1984):69. NC

### Liver Herbs, Additional Sources

#### BAICAL SKULLCAP

Amagaya, S., et al. "Treatment of chronic liver injury in mice by oral administration of xiao-chai-hu-tang." *J Ethnopharmacol* 25 (1989 2):181–187. NC

Chang, I.M., et al. "Plants with liver-protective activities, pharmacology and toxicology of aucubin." In: *Advances in Chinese Medicinal Material Research*. H.M. Chang, et al., eds. Philadelphia: World Scientific Press, 1984:269–285. NC

Choi, S.Y., et al. "Plants with liver protective activities." *Ann Rep Natl Prod Res Inst Seoul Natl Univ* 21 (1982):49–53. NC

Hong, N.D., et al. "Studies on the efficacy of combined preparations of crude drug (XL). Effect of sagan-tang on the central nervous, cardiovascular system and liver damage." *Korean J Pharmacog* 20 (1989)3:196–203. NC

Ihara, N., et al. "Protective effect of oriental crude drugs and kampo medicament on a fulminant type of galactosamine-induced hepatitis." *Wakanyaku shinpojumu (Kiroku)* 14 (1981):45–55. NC

Kato, M., et al. "Pharmacological studies on saiko-prescriptions. IV. Effect on liver injury induced by d-galactosamine in rats." *Yakugaku Zasshi* 104 (1984 7): 798–804. NC

Kim, J.S., et al. "Studies on the concurrent administrations of sosiho-tang extract and methionine. Effects on the liver lesion induced by carbon tetrachloride in rats." *Korean J Pharmacog* 17 (1986 2):148–152. NC

Kiso, Y., et al. "Antihepatotoxic actions of traditional Chinese medicines. The pharmacological interaction of components of a dai-saiko-to employing complement-mediated cytotoxicity in primary cultured mouse hepatocytes." *Phytother Res* 4 (1990 1):36–38. NC

Kumazawa, N., et al. "Protective effects of various methanol extracts of crude drugs on experimental hepatic injury induced by carbon tetrachloride in rats." *Yakugaku Zasshi* 110 (1990 12):950–957. NC

Lin, C.C., et al. "Hepatoprotective effect of the fractions of ban-zhi-lian on experimental liver injuries in rats." *J Ethnopharmacol* 56 (1997)3:193–200. NC

Um, K.J., et al. "Protective effects of a composite preparation (samulchungkantang) of crude drugs on hepatic injury induced by toxic drugs in rats." *Korean J Pharmacog* 26 (1995 4):390–410. NC

Yun, K.S., et al. "Liver protective activities of Korean medicinal plants." *Korean J Pharmacog* 11 (1980):149–152. NC

#### BOLDO

Bohm, K. "Choleretic action of some medicinal plants." *Arzneimittelforschung* 9 (1959):376–378. NC

Guerin, J.C., et al. "Antifungal activity of plant extracts used in therapy. I. Study of 41 plant extracts against 9 fungi species." *Ann Pharm Fr* 42 (1984 6):553–559. NC

Lanhers, M.C., et al. "Hepatoprotective and anti-inflammatory effects of a traditional medicinal plant of Chile, *Peumus boldus*." *Planta Med* 57 (1991 2):110–115. NC

Levy-Appert-Collin, M.C., and J. Levy. "Galenic preparations from the leaves of boldo." *J Pharm Belg* 32 (1977):13–. NC

Menghini, A., et al. "Antimicrobial activity on direct contact of certa in essential oils." *Plant Med Phytother* 21 (1987 1):36–42. NC

**BUPLEURUM**

Amagaya, S., et al. "Treatment of chronic liver injury in mice by oral administration of xiao-chai-hu-tang." *J Ethnopharmacol* 25 (1989 2):181–187. NC

Chiu, H.F., et al. "The pharmacological and pathological studies on several hepatic protective crude drugs from Taiwan." *Am J Chinese Med* 16 (1988 3–4):127–137. NC

Dan, L.K., et al. "Ultrastructural studies on the effect of 'gan fu kang' in preventing experimental liver damage in mice." *Chung I Tsa Chih* 8 (1988 2):151–154. NC

Goto, W., et al. "Suppression of hepatitis B virus surface antigen secretion by traditional plant medicines." *Phytother Res* 10 (1996 6):504–507. NC

Guinea, M.C., et al. "Biologically active triterpene saponins from bupleurum fruticosum." *Plant Med* 60 (1994 2):163–167. NC

Hong, N.D., et al. "Studies on the efficacy of combined preparations of crude drug (xl). Effect of sagan-tang on the central nervous and cardiovascular systems and liver damage." *Korean J Pharmacog* 20 (1989 3):196–203. NC

Kato, M., et al. "Pharmacological studies on saiko-prescriptions. IV. Effect on liver injury induced by d-galactosamine in rats." *Yakugaku Zasshi* 104 (1984 7):798–804. NC

Kim, J.S. "Studies on the concurrent administration of sosiho-tang extract and methionine. Effects on the liver lesion induced by carbon tetrachloride in rats." *Korean J Pharmacog* 17 (1986 2):148–152. NC

Kiso, Y., et al. "Antihepatotoxic actions of traditional Chinese medicines. The pharmacological interaction of components of a dai-saiko-to employing complement-mediated cytotoxicity in primary cultured mouse hepatocytes." *Phytother Res* 4 (1990 1):36–38. NC

Kumazawa, N., et al. "Protective effects of various methanol extracts of crude drugs on experimental hepatic injury induced by carbon tetrachloride in rats." *Yakugaku Zasshi* 110 (1990 12):950–957. NC

Lee, J.S., et al. "Pharmacologic activities of Saikosaponins. I. Effects on drug metabolizing enzymes modification and liver toxicities due to acetaminophen." *Korean J Pharmacog* 24 (1993 1):69–77. NC

———. "Pharmacologic activities of Saikosaponins. II. Effects of saikosaponin on metabolizing enzymes and lipid peroxide contents in liver." *Korean J Pharmacog* 24 (1993 2):153–158. NC

Lin, C.C., et al. "Hepatoprotective activity of Taiwan folk medicine: *Eclipta prostrata* Linn. against various hepatotoxins induced hepatotoxicity." *Phytomedicine* 3 (1996 2):155–161. NC

———. "Evaluation of hepatoprotective effects of 'chhit-chan-than' from Taiwan." *Int J Pharmacog* 33 (1995 2):139–143. NC

———. "Hepatoprotective effects of Taiwan folk medicine: *Ixeris chinensis* (Thunb.) NAK, on experimental liver injuries." *Am J Chinese Med* 22 (1994 3–4):243–254. NC

———. "Hepatoprotective effects of Taiwan folk medicine: *Wedelia chinensis* on three hepatotoxin induced hepatotoxicity." *Am J Chinese Med* 22 (1994 2):155–168. NC

Lin, C.C., et al. "The pharmacological and pathological studies on Taiwan folk medicine. III. The effects of *Bupleurum kaoi* and cultivated *Bupleurum falcatum* var. *komarowi*." *Am J Chinese Med* 18 (1990 3–4):105–112. NC

———. "The pharmacological and pathological studies on Taiwan folk medicine. III. The effects of *Echinops grijisii* and *E. latifolius*." Am J Chinese Med 18 (1990 3–4):113–120. NC

Lin, S.C., et al. "Protective and therapeutic effect of the Indonesian medicinal herb *Curcuma xanthorrhiza* on beta-d-galactosamine-induced liver disease." *Phytother Res* 10 (1996 2):131–135. NC

———. "Protective and therapeutic effects of *Curcuma xanthorrhiza* on hepatotoxin-induced liver damage." *Am J Chinese Med* 23 (1995 3–4):243–254. NC

———. "Hepatoprotective effects of Taiwan folk medicine: *Alternanthera sessilis* on liver damage induced by various hepatotoxins." *Phytother Res* 8 (1994 7):391–398. NC

Watanabe, A., et al. "Treatment of chronic hepatitis in elderly patients." *Int J Oriental Med* 14 (1989 1):57–62. NC

Yen, M.H., et al. "Anti-inflammatory and hepatoprotective activity of saikosaponin-f and the root extract of bupleurum root." *Fitoterapia 65* (1994 5):409–417. NC

**BURDOCK**

Brantner, A., et al. "Antibacterial activity of plant extracts used externally in traditional medicine." *J Ethnopharmacol* 44 (1994 1):35–40. NC

Chang, R.S. "Inhibition of growth of human immunodeficiency virus in vitro by crude extracts of Chinese medicinal herbs." *Antiviral Res* 9 (1988 3):163–175. NC

Collins, R.A. "A comparison of human immunodeficiency virus type 1 inhibition by partially purified aqueous extracts of Chinese medicinal herbs." *Life Sci* 60 (1997 23):345–351. NC

Costa, M. et al. "Screening in mice of some medicinal plants used for analgesic purposes in the state of Sao Paulo." *J Ethnopharmacol* 27 (1989 1/2):25–33. NC

Dombradi, C.A., et al. "Screening report on the antitumor activity of purified *Arctium lappa* extracts." *Tumori* 51 (1966):173–175. NC

Dornberger, K., et al. "Screening for antimicrobial and presumed cancerostatic plant metabolites." *Pharmazie* 37 (1982 3):215–221. NC

Goto, M., et al. "Uterus-contracting ingredients in plants." *Takeds Kenkyusho Nempo* 16 (1957):21–. NC

Ichikawa, K., et al. "CA-2+ antagonists from medicinal drugs." *J Pharmacobio Dyn* 10 (1987 3):49–. NC

Itokawa, H., et al. "Studies on the constituents of crude drugs having inhibitory activity against the contraction of the ileum caused by histamine or barium chloride (1). Screening test for the activity of commercially available crude drugs and the related plant materials." *Shoyakugaku Zasshi* 37 (1983 3):223–228. NC

Iwakami, S., et al. "Platelet activating factor (PAF) antagonists contained in medicinal plants: lignans and sesquiterpenes." *Chem Pharm Bull* 40 (1992 5):1196–1198; Son, K.H., et al. "Screening of platelet activating factor (PAF) antagonists from medicinal plants." *Korean J Pharmacog* 25 (1994 2):167–170. NC

Kim, S.Y., et al. "Antioxidant activities of selected oriental herb extracts." *J Am Oil Chem Soc* 71 (1994 6):633–640. NC

Koshimizu, K., et al. "Screening of edible plants against possible anti-tumor promoting activity." *Cancer Lett* 39 (1988 3):247–257; Foldeak, S., et al. "Tumor-growth inhibiting substances of plant origin. I. Isolation of the active principle of *Arctium lappa.*" *Acta Phys Chem* 10 (1964):91–93. NC

Lapinina, O.L. "Investigation of some plants to determine their sugar lowering action." *Farm Zh (Kiev).* 19 (1964 4):52–58. NC

Lin, C.C., et al. "Anti-inflammatory and radical scavenge effects of *Arctium lappa.*" *Am J Chinese Med* 24 (1996 2):127–137. NC

Makoru, L. Hair Restorer. Austrian patent # 176,950—1953. Also: Suzuki K, Hair Growth-Stimulating Preparations. Japanese patent: Japan Kokai Tokyo Koho-05 58,851, 1993. NC

Morita, K., et al. "A desmutagenic factor isolated from burdock (*Arctium lappa* Linne)." *Mutat Res* 129 (1984 1):25–31.

Oshima, Y., et al. "Anticomplementary activity of lignan-analogs of *Arctium lappa achenes.*" *Shoyakugaku Zasshi* 42 (1988 4):337–338. NC

Park, J.G., et al. "Antineoplastic effects of extracts from traditional medicinal plants." *Korean J Pharmacog* 24 (1993 3):223–230. NC

Sato, A. "Cancer chemotherapy with oriental medicine. I. Antitumor activity of crude drugs with human tissue cultures in in vitro screening." *Int J Orient Med* 15 (1990 4):171–183. NC

Silver, A.A., et al. "The effect of the ingestion of burdock root on normal and diabetic individuals. A preliminary survey." *Ann Intern Med* 5 (1931):274–. NC

Takeda, H., et al. "Correlation between the physical properties of dietary fibers and their protective activity against amaranth toxicity in rats." *J Nutr* 109 (1979):388–396. NC

Umehara, K., et al. "Studies on differentiation-inducers from *Arctium fructus.*" *Chem Pharm Bull* 41 (1993 10):1774–1779. NC

Yamaguchi, T., et al. "Desmutagenic activity of peroxidase on autodized linolenic acid." *Agr Biol Chem* 44 (1980 4):959–961. NC

Yang, K.S., et al. "Effect of *Arctii fructus* on low density lipoprotein oxidation." *Korean J Pharmacog* 28 (1997 4):275–279. NC

Yasukawa, K. et al. "Inhibitory effect of edible plant extracts on 12-0-tetradecanoylphorbol-13-acetate-induced ear oedema in mice." *Phytother Res* 7 (1993 2):185–189. NC

### DANDELION

Akhtar, M.S., et al. "Effects of *Portulaca oleracae* (Kulfa) and *Taraxacum officinale* (Dhudhal) in normoglycaemic and alloxan-treated hyperglycaemic rabbits." *J Pak Med Ass* 35 (1985):207–210. NC

Baba, K., et al. "Antitumor activity of hot water extracts of dandelion, *Taraxacum officinale,* correlation between antitumor activity and timing of administration." *Yakugaku Zasshi* 101 (1981):538–543. NC

Bohm, K. "Choleric action of some medicinal plants." *Arzneimittelforschung* 9 (1959):376–378. NC

Hobbs, Christopher. Taraxacum officinale: A Monograph and Literature Review. Eclectic Dispensatory. Sandy, OR: Eclectic Medical Publications, 1989. Multiple studies cited.

Horhammer, L. "Flavone concentration of medicinal plants with regard to their spasmolytic action." *Congr Sci Farm Conf Commun* 21st Pisa, 1961 21 (1962):578–588. NC

Jong, S.I. "The effect of Herba Taraxaci aqueous extract on experimental hypercholesterolemia." *Choson Minjujuui Inmin Konghwaguk Kwahagwon Tongbo* 1 (1996):48–50. NC

Kumazawa, N., et al. "Protective effects of various methanol extracts of crude drugs on experimental hepatic injury induced by carbon tetrachloride in rats." *Yakugaku Zasshi* 110 (1990 12):950–957. NC

Mars, Brigitte. *Dandelion Medicine.* Pownal, VT: Storey, 1999.

Mascolo, N., et al. "Biological screening of Italian medicinal plants for anti-inflammatory activity." *Phytother Res* 1 (1987 1):28–31. NC

Muto, Y., et al. "Studies on antiulcer agents. I. The effects of various methanol and aqueous extracts of crude drugs on antiulcer activity." *Yakugaku Zasshi* 114 (1994 2):980–994. NC

Racz-Kotilla, E., et al. "The action of *Taraxacum officinale* extracts on the body weight and diuresis of laboratory animals." *Planta Med* 26 (1974): 212–217.

Sekulic, D., et al. "Preliminary testing of plant extracts for acaricide activity." *Pharmazie* 50 (1995 12):835–. NC

Tita, B., et al. "*Taraxacum officinale* W.: Pharmacological effect of ethanol extract" Pharmacol Res 27 (1993 1):23–24. NC

Yasukawa, K., et al. "Inhibitory effects of edible plant extracts on 12-0-tetradecanoylphorbol-13-acetate-induced ear edema in mice." *Phytother Res* 7 (1993 2):185–189. NC

**MILK THISTLE**

Danielak, R., et al. "The preparation of vegetable products containing isofraxdin, silibin, and glaucium alkaloids and evaluation of their choleretic action." *Polish J Pharmacol Pharm* 25 (1973):271–283. NC

Flora, K., et al. "Milk thistle *(Silybum marianum)* for the therapy of liver disease." A*m J Gastroenterol* 93 (1998 2):139–143. NC

Gernandez, R., et al. "This is a preliminary report on the therapeutic assay of silimarini (legalon) in cholestasis of pregnancy, including twenty cases, plus twenty patients treated with placebo," *Rev Chil Obstet Ginecol* 41 (1982 1):22–29. NC

Hahn, Y.G. ,et al. "Zur Pharmakologie und Toxikologie von Silymarin des antihepatotoxisch Wirkprinzipes aus (L.) gaertin." *Arzneimittelforschung* 18 (1968 6):698–704. NC

Hobbs, Christopher. *Milk Thistle: The Liver Herb.* Loveland, CO: Interweave Press, 1998. Note: This is the best overall source on milk thistle, with nearly 100 citations; I have included in this section only the citations not present in his text.

Lend-Peschlow, E. "Properties and medical use of flavonolignans (Silymarin) from *Silybum marianum.*" *Phytother Res* 10 (1996):s25–s26. NC

Morazzoni, P., and E. Bombardelli. *"Silybum marianum (Carduus marianus)."* *Fitoterapia* 66 (1995 1):3–42. NC

Muriel, P., and M. Mourelle. "Prevention by silymarin of membrane alterations in acute $CCl_4$ liver damage." *J Appl Toxicol* 10 (1990 4):275–279. NC

Wang, M., et al. "Hepatoprotective properties of *Silybum marianum* herbal preparation on ethanol-induced liver damage." *Fitoterapia* 67 (1996 2):166–172. NC

Wei, B.F. "A clinical report on 39 cases of virus hepatitis treated with milk thistle *(Silybum marianum).*" *Chung Ts'ao Yao* 14 (1983 3):108–. NC

**PHYLLANTHUS**

Antarkar, D.S., et al. "A double-blind clinical trial of arogya-wardhani—an ayurvedic drug—in acute viral hepatitis." *Indian J Med Res* 72 (1990):588–593. NC

Bhaumik, A., et al. "Therapeutic efficacy of two herbal preparations in induced hepatopathy in sheep." *J Res Indian Med* 12 (1993 1):33–42. NC

Blumberg, B.S., et al. "Hepatitis B virus and hepatocellular carcinoma: treatment of HBV carriers with *Phyllanthus amarus.*" *Cancer Detect Prevent* 14 (1989):195–201. NC

Brook, M.G., et al. "Effect of *Phyllanthus amarus* on chronic carriers of hepatitis B virus." Lancet 8618 (1988):1017–1018. NC

Dixit, S.P., et al. "Bhumyamalaki (*Phyllanthus niruri*) and jaundice in children." *J Natl Integ Med Assoc* 25 (1983 8):269–272. NC

Gulati, R.K., et al. "Hepatoprotective studies on *Phyllanthus emblica* Linn. and quercetin." *Indian J Exp Biol* 33 (1995 4):261–268. NC

Lee, C.D., et al. "*Phyllanthus amarus* down regulates hepatitis B virus mRNA transcription and replication." *Eur J Clin Invest* 26 (1996 12):1069–1076. NC

Mehrotra, R., et al. "In vitro effect of *Phyllanthus amarus* on hepatitis B virus." *Indian J Med Res* 93 (1991 2):71–73. NC

Ott, M., et al. "*Phyllanthus amarus* suppresses hepatitis B virus by interrupting interactions between HBV enhancer 1 and cellular transcription factors." *Eur J Clin Invest* 27 (1997 11):908–915. NC

Rao, Y.S. "Experimental production of liver damage and its protection with *Phyllanthus niruri* and *Capparis spinosa* (both ingredients of LIV-52) in white albino rats." *Probe* 24 (1985 2):117–119. NC

Roy, A.K., et al. "*Phyllanthus emblica* fruit extract and ascorbic acid modify hepatotoxic and renotoxic effects of metals in mice." *Int J Pharmacog* 29 (1991)2:117–126. NC

Sama, S.K., et al. "Efficacy of an indigenous compound preparation (LIV-52) in acute viral hepatitis: a double blind study." *Indian J Med Res* 64 (1976):738–. NC 19. Munshi, A., et al. "Evaluation of anti-hepadnavirus activity of *Phyllanthus amarus* and Phyllanthus maderaspatensis in duck hepatitis B virus carrier Pekin ducks." *J Med Virol* 41 (1993 4):275–281. NC

Sane, R.T., et al. "Hepatoprotection by *Phyllanthus amarus and Phyllanthus debilis* in CCl$_4$-induced liver dysfunction." Curr Sci 68 (1995 12):1243–1246. NC

Syamasundar, K.V., et al. "Antihepatotoxic principles of *Phyllanthus niruri* herb." *J Ethnopharmacol* 14 (1985 1):41–44. NC

Thabrew, M.R. "Phytogenic agents in the therapy of liver disease." *Phytother Res* 10 (1996 6):461–467. NC

Thyagarajan, S.P., et al. "Effect of *Phyllanthus amarus* on carriers of hepatitis B virus." Lancet 8614 (1988):764–766. NC

Thyagarajann, S.P., et al. "*Phyllanthus amaras* and hepatitis B." Lancet 336 (1990 8720):949–950. NC

Umarani, D., et al. "Ethanol induced metabolic alterations and the effect of *Phyllanthus niruri* in their reversal." *Ancient Life Sci* 4 (1985 3):174–180. NC

Unander, D.W., et al. "Usage and bioassays in Phyllanthus (Euphorbiaceae). IV. Clustering of antiviral uses and other effects." *J Ethnopharmacol* 45 (1995 1):1–18. NC

## PICRORHIZA

Ansari, R.A., et al. "Antihepatotoxic properties of picroliv: an active fraction from rhizomes of *Picrorrhiza kurroa.*" *J Ethnophamacol* 34 (1991 1): 61–68. NC

Ansari, R.A. et al. "Hepatoprotective activity of kitkin. The iridoid glycoside mixture of *Picrorrhiza kurroa*." *Indian J Med Res* 87 (1988 4):401–404. NC

Antarkar, D.S., et al. "A double-blind clinical trial or arogya-wardhani—an ayurvedic drug—in acute viral hepatitis." *Indian J Med Res* 72 (1980):588–593. NC

Aswal, R.S., et al. "Extraction of a hepato-protective fraction containing picroside I and kutkoside from *Picrorrhiza kurroa*." Patent US-5,145,955. 1992. NC

Chang, I.M., et al. "Plants with liver-protective activities, pharmacology and toxicology of aucubin." In: *Advances in Chinese Medicinal Materials Research*. H.M. Chang, et al., editors. Philadelphia: World Scientific Press; 1984.

Choi, S.Y., et al. "Plants with liver-protective activities."*Ann Rep Nat Prod Res Inst Seoul Natl Univ* 21 (1982):49–53. NC

Dorsch, W., et al. "Antiasthmatic effects of *Picrorrhiza kurroa*: Androsin prevents allergen- and PAF-induced bronchial obstruction in guinea pigs." *Int Arch Allergy Appl Immunol* 95 (1981):128–133.

Dwivedi, Y., et al. "Perfusion with picroliv reverses biochemical changes induced in livers of rats toxicated with galactosamine or thioacetamide." *Planta Med* 59 (1993 5): 418–420.

———. "Picroliv protects against aflatoxin B1 acute hepatotoxicity in rats." *Pharmacol Res* 27 (1993 2):189–199. NC

———. "Effects of picroliv, the active principle of *Picrorrhiza kurroa*, on biochemical changes in rat liver poisoned by *Amanita phalloides*." *Chung-kuo Yao Li Hseuh Pao* 13 (1992 3):197–200. NC

———. "Picroliv affords protection against thioacetamide-induced hepatic damage in rats." *Planta Med* 57 (1991)1:25–28.

———. "Picroliv protects against monocrotaline-induced hepatic damage in rats." *Pharmacol Res* 23 (1991 4):399–407. NC

———. "Prevention of paracetamol-induced hepatic damage in rats by picroliv, the standardized active fraction from *Picrorrhiza kurroa*." *Phytother Res* 5 (1991 3):115–119. NC

Kapahi, B.K., et al. "Description of *Picrorrhiza kurroa*, a source of the Ayurvedic drug kutaki." *Ind J Pharmacog* 31 (1993):217–222.

Lin, C.C., et al. "Evaluation of hepato-protective activity of picroliv (from *Picrorrhiza kurroa*) in *Mastomys natalensis* infected with *Plasmodium berghei*." *Indian J Med Res* 92 (1990 1):34–37. NC

Rastogi, R. et al. "Effect of picroliv on impaired hepatic mixed-function oxidase system in $CCl_4$ intoxicated rats." *Drug Develop Res* 41 (1997 1):44–47. NC

———. "Effect of picroliv on antioxidant-system in liver of rats, after partial hepatectomy." *Phytother Res* 9 (1995 5):364–367. NC

Saksena, S., et al. "Rifampicin induced hepatotoxicity in rat: protective effect of picroliv." *Drug Dev Res* 33 (1994 1):46–50.

Saraswat, B., et al. "Hepatoprotective effect of picroliv against rifampicin-induced toxicity." *Drug Develop Res* 40 (1997 4):299–303. NC

Sharma, M.L. et al. "Immunostimulatory effect of Picrorrhiza extract." *J Ethnopharmacol* 41 (1994):185–192.

Singh, D.D., et al. "A comparative study of Ayurvedic drugs *Picrorrhiza kurroa* (Kutaki) and *Berberis aristata* (Daru Haridra) in acute viral hepatitis at Varanasi (India)." *J Res Edu Ind Med* 10 (1991)4:1–4. NC

Singh, N., et al. "Indian plants as anti-stress agents." Abstr Internati Rees Cong Nat Prod Coll Pharm Univ N Carolina. Chapel Hill, NC, July 7–12, 1985. Abstract 202, 1985. NC

Srivastava, S. et al. "Effect of picroliv on liver regeneration in rats." *Fitoterapia* 67 (1996 3):252–256. NC

Tripathi, S.C., et al. "Hepatoprotective activity of pircoliv against alcohol-carbon tetrachloride induced liver damage in rats." *Indian J Pharmacy* 23 (1991 3):143–148. NC

Vaishwanar, I., et al. "Effect of two Ayurvedic drugs Shilajeet and Eclinol on changes in liver and serum lipids produced by carbon tetrachloride" *Indian J Exp Biol* 14 (1976 1):57–58. NC

Visen, P.K.S., et al. "Prevention of galactosamine-induced hepatic damage by picroliv: study on bile flow and isolated hepatocytes (ex vivo)." *Planta Med* 59 (1993 1):37–41. NC

———. "Hepatoprotective activity of picroliv isolated from *Picrorrhiza kurroa* against thioacetamide toxicity on rat hepatocytes." *Phytother Res* 5 (1991 5):224–227. NC

Yun, H.S., et al. "Liver protective activities of Korean medicinal plants." *Korean J Pharmacog* 11 (1990):149–152. NC

**REISHI**

Aoki, M., et al. "Antiviral substances with systemic effects produced by basidiomycetes such as *Fomes fomentarius.*" *Biosci Biotech Biochem* 57 (1993 2):278–282. NC

Byuh, S.H., and I.H. Kim. "Studies on the concurrent administration of medicines (VII). Effects of concurrent administration of *Ganoderma lucidum* extract and glutathione on the liver damage induced by carbon tetrachloride in rats." *Yahak Hoe Chi* 31 (1987 3):13–139. NC

Chen, W.C., et al. "Effects of *Ganoderma lucicum* and Krestin on subset T-cell in spleen of gamma-irradiated mice" *Am J Chinese Med* 23 (1995 3/4):189–198. NC

Cheng, Z.H., et al. "Effects of Lingzhi *(Ganoderma lucidum)* on hemorrheology parameters and symptoms of hypertensive patients with hyperlipidemia and sequelae of cerebral thrombosis." *J Chin Pharm Sci* 1 (1992 1):46–50. NC

Chiajumrus, S., et al. "Purification and characterization of antitumor polysaccharides isolated from fruiting body and mycelium of *Ganoderma lucidum.*" *Util Renewable Resour* 9 (1996):271–281. NC

Goto, W., et al. "Suppression of hepatitis B virus surface antigen secretion by traditional plant medicines." *Phytother Res* 10 (1996 6):504–507. NC

Hobbs, Christopher. *Medicinal Mushrooms.* Loveland, CO: Interweave Press, 1996. One of the best looks at scientific studies and active constituents.

Ito, H., et al. "Activation of reticuloendothelial system by antitumor polysaccharide from *Ganoderma lucidum.*" *Igaku to Seibutsugaku* 127 (1993 5):345–348. NC

Jeong, H. "Studies on the anticomplementary activity of Korean higher fungi." *Han'guk Kyunhakhoe Chi* 18 (1990 3):145–148. NC

Kabir, Y., et al. "Dietary effect of *Ganoderma lucidum* mushroom on blood pressure and lipid levels in spontaneously hypertensive rats." *J Nutr Sci Vitamiol* 34 (1988 4):433–438. NC

Kim, D.H., et al. "Beta-glucuronidase-inhibitory activity and hepatoprotective effect of *Ganoderma lucidum.*" *Biol Pharm Bull* 22 (1999 2):162–164. NC

Lee, M.J., and M.H. Chung. "Effect of *Ganoderma lucidum* extract on experimentally induced hepatic damage and hyperlipidemic rats." *Korean J Pharmacog* 18 (1987 4):254–264. NC

Lei, L.S., and Z.B. Lin. "Effects of *Ganoderma polysaccharides* on the activity of DNA polymerase alpha of splenocytes and immune function in aged mice." *Yao Hsueh Hsueh Pao* 28 (1993 8):577–582. NC

Lin, J.M., et al. "Radical scavenger and antihepatotoxic activity of *Ganoderma formosanum, Ganoderma lucidum,* and *Ganoderma neo-japonicum.*" *J Ethnopharmacol* 47 (1995 1):33–41. NC

———. "Evaluation of the anti-inflammatory and liver-protective effects of *Anoectochilus formosanus, Ganoderma lucidum,* and *Gynostemma pentaphyllum* in rats." *Am J Chinese Med* 21 (1993 1):59–69. NC

Liu, G.T., et al. "A comparison of the protective actions of biphenyl dimethyldicarboxylate trans-stilbene, alcoholic extracts of *Fructus schizandrae* and *Ganoderma lucidum* against experimental liver injury in mice." *Yao Hsueh Hsueh Pao* 14 (1979):598–604. NC

———. "Some pharmacological actions of *Ganoderma lucidum* and *G. japonicum* of mouse liver." *Yao Hsueh Hsueh Pao* 14 (1979 5):284–287. NC

Park, E.J., et al. "Antifibrotic effects of a polysaccharide extracted from Ganoderma lucidum, glycyrrhizin, and pentoxifylline in rats with cirrhosis induced by biliary obstruction." *Biol Pharm Bull* 20 (1997 4):417–420. NC

———. "The antifibrotic effects of polysaccharides extracted from *Ganoderma lucidum* on experimental hepatic cirrhosis." *Yahak Hoe Chi* 38 (1994 3):338–344. NC

Shin, H.W., et al. "Studies on inorganic composition and immunopotentiating activity of *Ganoderma lucidum* in Korea." *Korean J Pharmacog* 16 (1985 4):181–190. NC

Teow, S.S. "The therapeutic value of *Ganoderma lucidum.*" Fifth International Mycological Conference Abstracts. Vancouver, B.C. August 14–21, 1994. NC

Wang, S.Y., et al. "The anti-tumor effect of *Ganoderma lucidum* is mediated by cytokines released from activated macrophages and T lymphocytes." *Int J Cancer* 70 (1997 6):699–705. NC

Willard, Terry. *Reishi Mushroom.* Seattle, WA: Sylvan Press, 1990. Provides extensive information.

Yan, R., et al. "Treatment of chronic hepatitis B with Wulingdan Pill." *Journal of the Fourth Military Medical College of Chinese People's Liberation Army* 10 (1987):183–185. NC

Yanfg, L.L., et al. "Antihepatotoxic actions of Formosan plant drugs." *J Ethnopharmacol* 19 (1987 1):103–110. NC

## TURMERIC

Aruna, K. "Anticarcinogenic effects of some Indian plant products." *Food Chem Toxicol* 30 (1992 11):953–956. NC

Bonte, F., et al. "Protective effect of curcuminoids on epidermal skin cells under free oxygen radical stress." *Planta Med* 63 (1997 3):265–266. NC

Cai, D.F., et al. "Anti-viral and interferon-inducing effect of kangli powder." *Chung Hsi I Chieh Ho Tsa Chih* 8 (1988 12):731–733. NC

Cherdchu, C. et al. "Cobra neurotoxin inhibition activity found in extract of *Curcuma* spp. (Zingiberaceae)." *J Med Assoc Thai* 57 (1991):1–7.

Chuthaputti, A., et al. "Anti-inflammatory activity of *Curcuma longa* Linn. Rhizomes." *Bull Dept Med Sci* 36 (1994 4):197–209. NC

Desphande, S.S., et al. "Chemoprotective efficacy of curcumin-free aqueous turmeric extract in 7,12-dimethylbenz[a]anthracene-induced rat mammary tumorigenesis." *Cancer Lett* 123 (1998 1):35–40. NC

———. "Inhibitory effects of curcumin-free aqueous turmeric extract on benzo[a]pyrene-induced forestomach papillomas in mice." *Cancer Lett* 118 (1997 1):79–85. NC

Dixit, V.P. "Hypolipidaemic effects of *Curcuma longa* L. and *Nardostachys jatamansi* D.C. in triton-induced hyperlipidaemic rats." *Indian J Physiol Pharmacol* 32 (1988 4):299–304. NC

Godhwani, J.L., et al. "Modification of immunological response by garlic, gugal, and turmeric: an experimental study in animals." Abstr 12th Ann Conf Indian Pharmacol Soc. Jammu-Tawi, India, September 30–October 2, 1980. NC

Goto, W., et al. "Suppression of hepatitis B virus surface antigen secretion by traditional plant medicines." *Phyto Res* 10 (1996 6):504–507. NC

Hikino, H. "Antihepatoxic activity of crude drugs." *Yakugaku Zasshi* 105 (1985 2):109–118. NC

Jain, J.P., et al. "Clinical trials of haridra (*Curcuma longa*) in cases of tamak swasa (bronchial asthma) and kasa (bronchitis)." *J Res Indian Med Yoga Homeopathy* 14 (1979 2):110–119. NC

Joyeux, M. et al. "Screening of antiradical, antilipoperoxidant, and hepatoprotective effects of nine plant extracts used in Caribbean folk medicine." *Phytother Res* 9 (1995 3):228–230. NC

Kinoshita, G., et al. "Immunological studies on polysaccharide reactions from crude drugs." *Shoyakugaku Zasshi* 40 (1986 3):325–332. NC

Kiso, Y., et al. "Antihepatotoxic principles of *Curcuma longa* rhizomes." *Planta Med* 49 (1983 3):185–187. NC

———. "Liver-protective drugs. The validity of oriental medicines. Application of carbon tetrachloride-induced liver lesion in mice for screening of liver protective crude drugs." *Shoyakugaku Zasshi* 36 (1982): 238–244. NC

Kosuge, T., et al. "Studies on antitumor activities and antitumor principles of Chinese herbs. I. Antitumor activities of Chinese herbs." *Yakugaku Zasshi* 105 (1985 8):791–795. NC

Kumar, A., et al. "Efficacy of some indigenous drugs in tissue repair in buffaloes." *Indian Vet J* 70 (1993 1):42–44. NC

Kuttan, R., et al. "Potential anticancer activity of turmeric (*Curcuma longa*)." *Cancer Lett* 29 (1985 2):197–202. NC

Lin, S.C. "Protective and therapeutic effects of *Curcuma xanthorrhiza* on hepatotoxin-induced liver damage." *Am J Chinese Med* 23 (1995 3/4):243–254. NC

Liu, Y.G. "Hypolipemics and blood platelet aggregation inhibitors comprising fish oil and plant extracts." Patent. US-4,842,859, 1989. NC

Miquel, J., et al. "Effects of turmeric on blood and liver lipoperoxide levels of mice." *Age* 18 (1995 4):171–174. NC

Mukundan, M.A., et al. "Effect of turmeric and curcumin on BP-DNA adducts." *Carcinogenesis* 14 (1993 3):493–496. NC

Ozaki, Y., et al. "Cholagogic effect of Zingiber plants obtained from Indonesia." *Shoyakygaku Zasshi* 42 (1988 4):333–336. NC

Prucksunand, C., et al. "Prevention action of turmeric against HCL-induced gastric necrosis in rats." *Thai J Pharm Sci* 21 (1997 1):43–48. NC

Selvam, R., et al. "The anti-oxidant activity of turmeric (*Curcuma longa*)." *J Ethnopharmacol* 47 (1995 2):59–67. NC

Shalini, V.K., et al. "Lipid peroxide induced DNA damage: protection by turmeric (*Curcuma longa*)." *Mol Cell Biochem* 77 (1987 1):3–10. NC

Shimizu, S., et al. "Inhibitory effect of curcumin on fatty acid desaturation in *Mortierella alpina* 1S-4 and rat liver microsomes." *Lipids* 27 (1992 7):509–512. NC

Singh, A., et al. "Postnatal modulation of hepatic biotransformation system enzymes via translactational exposure of F1 mouse pups to turmeric and curcumin." *Chem Lett* 96 (1995):87–93. NC

Snow, Joanne Marie. "*Curcuma longa* L. (Zingiberaceae)." *Protocol Journal of Botanic Medicine*. 1 (1995 2):43–46. Cites multiple studies and journals.

Soni, K.B. "Protective effect of food additives on aflatoxin-induced mutagenicity and hepatocarcinogenicity." *Chem Lett* 115 (1997 2):129–13. NC

———. "Inhibition of aflatoxin-induced liver damage in ducklings by food additives." *Mycotoxin Res* 9 (1993 1):22–27. NC

———. "Effect of oral curcumin administration on serum peroxides and cholesterol levels in human volunteers." *Indian J Physiol Pharmacol* 36 (1992):273–275.

———. "Reversal of aflatoxin induced liver damage by turmeric and curcumin." *Cancer Lett* 66 (1992 2):115–121. NC

Soudamini, K.K., et al. "Chemoprotective effect of curcumin against cyclophosphamide toxicity." *Indian J Pharm Sci* 54 (1992 6):213–217. NC

Thamlikitkul, V., et al. "Randomized double blind study of *Curcuma domestica* Val. for dyspepsia." *J Med Assoc Thailand* 72 (1989 11):613–620. NC

Toda, S., et al. "Natural antioxidants. III. Antioxidative components isolated from rhizome of *Curcuma longa* L." *Chem Pharm Bull* 33 (1985 4):1725–1728. NC

Yaksukawa, K. et al. "Inhibitory effect of edible plant extracts on 12-0-tetradecanoylphorbol-13-acetate-induced ear oedema in mice" *Phytother Res* 7 (1993 2):185–189. NC

Yano, S.G., et al. "Antiallergenic activity of *Curcuma longa*: active principles and mode of action." *Wakan Iyakugaku Zasshi* 12 (1995 4):269–272. NC

## The Liver, Viral Hepatitis, Hepatitis C

Askari, Fred. *Hepatitis C: The Silent Epidemic*. New York: Plenum Press, 1999.

Bader, Teddy. *Viral Hepatitis: Practical Evaluation and Treatment*. Seattle: Hogrefe and Huber, 1997.

Bergner, Paul. "Licorice as a liver herb." *Medical Herbalism* 6 (1994 1):6–7.

———. "Milk thistle in Eclectic medical practice." *Medical Herbalism* 6 (1994 1):5.

———. "Herbal treatment of functional liver disease." *Medical Herbalism* 5 (1993 4):1–5.

Boyle, Wade. "Dueling liver botanicals" *Medical Herbalism* 4 (1992 2):1,10.

Cabrera, Chanchal. "Milk thistle: a clinician's report" *Medical Herbalism* 6 (1994 1):1–4.

Davis, Robert. "Millions hit hepatitis C deadline: as silent killer roars, medical science struggles to find response." *USA Today*. 8 June 1999:D1.

———. "Silent tenacious killer ravages the liver: with no cure and little treatment, hepatitis C is the topic of discussion for international symposium." *USA Today*. 8 June 1999:D6.

Everson, G., and Hedy Weinberg. *Living With Hepatitis C: A Survivor's Story*. New York: Hatherleigh Press, 1998.

Fackelmann, Kathleen. "Hepatitis C behind bars: deadly liver disease could break out as infected prisoners go home." *USA Today*. 19 October 1999: D1.

———. "Lack of drugs puts inmates on death row." *USA Today*. 19 October 1999:D9.

———. "Long after wars are over, veterans battle hepatitis C." *USA Today.* 19 October 1999:D9.

Feldman, M., and B. Scharschmidt and M. Sleisenger. *Gastrointestinal and Liver Disease.* Philadelphia:W.B. Saunders Company, 1998.

Holmes, E.C., et al. "An RNA virus tree of life." In: *Evolution of Microbial Life.*

Johnson, A., and David Triger. *Liver Disease and Gallstones.* Oxford: Oxford University Press, 1992.

Roberts, D. McL, et al., editors. Fifty-fourth Symposium of the Society for General Microbiology, March 1996. London: Cambridge University Press, 1996.

Roybal, Beth. *Hepatitis C: A Personal Guide to Good Health.* Berkeley, CA: Ulysses Press, 1997.

Simmonds, P. "Evolution of hepatitis C virus." In: *Evolution of Microbial Life.*

Specter, Steven, ed. *Viral Hepatitis: Diagnosis, Therapy and Prevention.* Totowa, NJ: Humana Press, 1999.

Stansbury, Jill. "Four cases of hepatitis C." *Medical Herbalism* 6 4:1–7, 1994.

Tilgner, Sharol. "Liver: sluggish or damaged." *Medical Herbalism* 5 (1993 4):4.

Tizard, Ian. *Immunology: An Introduction.* Philadelphia: W.B. Saunders, 1988.

Turkington, Carol. *Hepatitis C: The Silent Killer.* Chicago: Contemporary Books, 1998.

## Nutritional Supplements, Additional Sources

Bergner, Paul. *The Healing Power of Minerals, Special Nutrients, and Trace Elements.* Rocklin, CA: Prima Publishing; 1997.

Berkson, Burt. *The Alpha Lipoic Acid Breakthrough.* Rocklin, CA: Prima Publishing; 1998. Contains numerous journal citations.

Sosin, Allan, and B.L. Jacobs. *Alpha Lipoic Acid: Nature's Ultimate Antioxidant.* New York: Kensington; 1998. Contains numerous citations.

Watson, Cynthia. *All about Alpha-Lipoic Acid.* New York: Avery; 1999.

## Other Herbs Successful in Human Trials for Treatment of Hepatitis

A combination mixture of fresh leaf of *Citrus reticulata, Astragalus membranaceus, Smilax china, gardenia jasminoides, Pueraria lobata, Curcuma aromatica, Glycyrrhiza glabra,* and *Vigna sinensis.* Kang, L.S., et al. "Treatment of 120 cases of hepatitis B with hepatitis B mixture." *Shanxi J Traditional Chinese Med* 3 (1987 6):16–17. NC

*Berberis aristata:* Singh, D.S., et al. "A comparative study of Ayurvedic drugs *Picrorhiza kurroa* and *Berberis aristata* in acute viral hepatitis at Varanasi (India)." *J Res Edu Ind Med* 10 (1991 4):1–4. NC

*Carduus nutans:* Cristea, E., et al. "Medicine with hepatoprotective activity." Patent. Rom-71,851, 1980. NC

*Cochlospermum planchonii:* Wolga, J. "*Cochlospernum planchonii* extracts, a method for their preparation and their hepatoprotective properties." Patent. Eur patent application 300,887, 1989. NC

Combination mixture of *Achillea millefolium, Capparis spinosa, Cassia occidentalis, Cichorium intybus, Solanum nigrum, Tamarix gallica,* and *Terminalia arjuna:* Sama, S.K., et al. "Efficacy of an indigenous compound preparation (LIV-52) in acute viral hepatitis: a double-blind study." *Eur J Clin Invest* 27 (1997 11):908–915. NC

Combination mixture of *Gardenia jasminoides, Angelica sinensis, Atractylodes macrocephala, Paeonia albiflora, Salvia miltiorrhiza, Artemisia scoparia, Astragalus membranaceus, Rehmannia glutinosa, Paeonia moutan,* and *Poria cocos:* Han, J., and F. Li. "Clinical observations on the efficacy of qiang gan ruan jian tang in the treatment of 105 cases of uncompensated cirrhosis of the liver" *Natl Med J China* 59 (1979):584–588. NC

*Cotinus coggygria:* Zhang, Z.C., et al. "Antihepatitis component of *Continus coggygria.*" *Chung Yao T'ung Pao* 13 (1988 3):34–35. NC

*Eclipta alba:* "A trial of Bhringaraja Ghanasatwavati on the patients of Kostha-shakhasrita Kamala (with special reference to hepatocellular jaundice)." *J Natl Integ Med Assoc* 24 (1982 9):265–269. NC

*Paeonia rubra:* Wang, C. "Comparison of jaundice-reducing effects of drugs for eliminating pathogenic heat from the blood and invigorating blood circulation, corticosteroids, and toxic heat-removing drugs in treatment of cholestatic hepatitis." *Chin J Integ Trad West Med* 4 (1984 2):80–85. NC

*Polyporus umbellatus:* Yang, S.C., et al. "Clinical and experimental research on *Ployporus umbellatus* polysaccharide in the treatment of chronic viral hepatitis." *Chung Hsi I Chieh Ho Tsa Chih* 8 (1988 3):141–143. NC

*Rheum officinale:* Wu, C., et al. "A preliminary analysis of the effects of single *Rheum officinale* with heavy doses in the treatment of acute icteric hepatitis." *Chin J Integ Trad West Med* 4 (1984 2):88–89. NC

*Sedum sarmentosum:* Ding, G.S. "Trials of some Chinese medicinal herbs." Proceedings of the U.S.-China Pharmacology Symposium. October 29–31, 1979 (National Academy of Sciences, 1980, 103–121.) NC

*Symphytum officinale:* Hirosaki, K. "Comfrey extracts for treatment of liver cirrhosis." Patent. Japan Kokai Tokyo Koho-78 127, 811, 1978. NC

# INDEX

Entries in **bold** indicate recipes; page references in **bold** indicate boxes.

## A

Abdominal bloating, 22, 99
Acetaminophen, 84
*Achillea millefolium,* 53
AIDS. *See* HIV
Albumin, 19, 112
Alcohol extractions, 116
Alcoholic beverages
   adverse reaction to, 2, 99
   limiting consumption of, 90, 92,
     94, 98, 101
Allergies, 2
Alpha-lipoic acid (ALA), **77,** 76–78,
   98
ALT/AST tests, 112
Amino acids, 19–20
*Anemone pusitilla,* 100
*Angelica sinensis,* 53, 100
Antibodies, 15
Antibody detection test, 111
Apoptosis, 11
Appetite, loss of, 101
Armpits, swelling under, 101
*Artemisia scoparia,* 53
Artichokes, 90, 94
*Articum lappa. See* Burdock
Ascites, 22, 99
Ashwagandha *(Withania som-*
   *nifera),* **55,** 55–57, 97–101
   contraindications, 57
   preparation/dosage, 56
Asian ginseng. *See* Panax (or Asian)
   ginseng

Astragalus *(Astralagus membrana-*
   *ceous),* 53, **55,** 57–59, 98, 100
   contraindications, 59
   preparation/dosage, 58
   recipes, 60, 95
*Atractylodes macrocephala,* 54
Attention deficit disorder, 101

## B

Baical skullcap *(Scutellaria baicalen-*
   *sis),* **24,** 25–26
   contraindications, 26
   preparation/dosage, 26
   uses of, 25–26, 99, 100, 101
Beets, 90, 94, 95
*Berberis aristata,* 52
Beverages, 89–92, 100
Bile, 17–18
Bile ducts, 2, 16–17, 21
Bile pigments, 17
Bile salts, 17–18
Bilirubin, 17, 112
Blackberry leaf *(Rubus villosus),* 100
Black cohosh *(Cimifuga racemosa),*
   100
Bladderwrack *(Fucus vesculosus, F.*
   *distichus),* 84–85, 99
Blood
   filtered by liver, 16, 21–22
   HCV spread by infected, 2, 5–6
   hemolysis, 3
Blood fat levels, test for, 112
Blood sugar disorders, 20, 99

Blood tests, 97, 111–112

Boldo *(Peumus boldus)*, **24,** 27–28, 99, 101
  contraindications, 28
  preparation/dosage, 28
  uses of, 27–28

Boneset *(Eupatorium perfoliatum)*, **55,** 50–61, 92, 100
  contraindications, 61
  preparation/dosage, 60–61

Botanical medicines for HCV and liver, 23–53. *See also* Herbal medicines, making/using; *specific herbs*
  descriptions of herbs, 25–53
  overview, 23–24
  types of actions, 24

Botanical support for immune system, 22, 54–75. *See also specific herbs*
  descriptions of herbs, 55–75
  in hepatitis protocols, 97–98
  qualities of immune-boosting herbs, 54–55

Brain fog, 101

Bread, 93

Bruises, 17

Bupleurum *(Bupleurum chinense or B. falcatum, B. fruticosum, B. kaoi)*, **25,** 28–31
  contraindications, 31
  preparation/dosage, 31
  uses of, 29–31, 97, 98, 100, 101

Burdock *(Articum lappa)*, **25,** 31–34
  contraindications, 34

  preparation/dosage, 33
  recipes, 95, 117
  uses of, 32–33, 90, 97, 98, 99, 100, 101

### C
Caffeine, 90

*Camellia sinensis,* 87–88

Cancer, liver, 100

*Capparis spinosa,* 53

Capsules, 117
  ashwagandha, 56
  astralagus, 58
  baical skullcap, 26
  bladderwrack, 85
  boldo, 28
  bupleurum, 31
  burdock, 33
  codonopsis, 63
  dandelion, 37
  licorice, 65
  milk thistle, 40
  phyllanthus, 43
  picrorhiza, 45
  red root, 69
  schizandra, 71
  Siberian ginseng, 72
  tienchi ginseng, 75
  turmeric, 51

Carbohydrate conversion by liver, 19

*Carduus nutans,* 52

Carmoviruses, 11

*Cassia occidentalis,* 53

*Ceanothus* spp. *See* Red root

Chest pains, palpitations, 99

Children
  dosages for, 118
  hepatitis A, 4
  hepatitis B, 6
Chills, intermittent, 100
*Chionanthus virginica,* 101
Chlorella *(Chlorella pyrendoidosa),*
    85–87, 89, 93, 99
  contraindications, 87
  preparation/dosage, 87
Cholestasis, 94
Cholesterol
  high, 20, 100
  tests for, 112
Chronic fatigue, 2, 4, 18–21, 100
*Cichorium intybus,* 53
*Cimifuga racemosa,* 100
Cirrhosis, 2, 21–22, 100
*Citrus riticulata,* 53
*Cochlospermum planchonii,* 52
Codonopsis (*Codonopsis pilosula,*
    et al.), **55,** 61–63, 97–101
  contraindications, 63
  preparation/dosage, 62–63
Cognitive dysfunction, 101
**Combination Tincture Formula
    for the Liver,** 117
Comfrey *(Symphytum officinale),* 52
Cooking methods, 93
*Cotinus coggygria,* 52
Culver's root *(Leptandra virginica),*
    101
*Curcuma aromatica,* 53
*Curcuma longa. See* Turmeric

**D**

Dandelion *(Taraxacum officinale),*
    **24,** 34–37

  contraindications, 37
  preparation/dosage, 36–37
  recipes, 117
  uses of, 35–36, 90, 97–101
Decoctions, 48, 52–53, 69, 71, 115
Depression, 2, 3, 18–19, 100, 101
Devil's root bark *(Oplopanax hor-
    ridum),* 99
Diarrhea, 3, 4, 100
Diet, 83–95
  hepatitis A, 4
  in hepatitis protocols, 98
  recommended foods, 83–89, 94
  ten-week low-fat cleansing diet,
    89–95
Dizziness, 100
DNA
  HCV b-DNA test, 113
  hepatitis B and, 6
  viruses and, 104–105, 107
Dolan, Matthew, 22
Dong quai *(Angelica sinensis),* 53,
    100

**E**

Ebola Zaire virus, 102
Echinacea, 100
*Eclipta alba,* 52
*Eleutherococcus senticosus.See*
    Siberian ginseng
Enzymes, 20
Epstein-Barr virus, 9, 107,
    109–110
*Eupatorium perfoliatum.See*
    Boneset
Exhaustion. *See* Chronic fatigue
Extremities, numbness in, 101

## F

Fats
    aversion to fatty foods, 2, 99
    blood fat levels, tests for, 112
    breakdown by liver, 20, 83
    low-fat diet, 89–95, 98
Fever, intermittent, 100
Flaviviridae, 11
Flaviviruses, 11
Fluid retention, 2, 21, 99
Flulike illness, 2, 3, 100
Fringetree bark (Chionanthus vir-
        ginica), 101
Fruits, 90, 100
Fucus vesculosus, F. distichus,
        84–85

## G

Gallbladder, 16–18
Ganoderma lucidum. See Reishi
Gardenia jasminoides, 53
Garlic, 90, 94, 95, 100
Gentian, 100
Ginger, 92, 95, 100, 101
Ginkgo (Ginkgo bilboa), 100, 101
Ginseng. See Panax (or Asian) gin-
        seng; Siberian ginseng;
        Tienchi ginseng
Glucose, 19
Glutathione, 20
Glycerites, 118–119
Glycogen, 19
Glycyrrhiza glabra.See Licorice
Grain, 89–90, 98
Green tea (Camellia sinensis),
        87–88, 90, 100, 101
Groin, swelling in, 101

## H

Hair, loss of, 21
Hantavirus, 106
HCV b-DNA test, 113
HDL (high-density lipoprotein),
        20, 112
Hemolysis, 3
Hepaciviruses, 11
Hepatitis A virus, 4, 11
Hepatitis B virus, 6
Hepatitis C Handbook, The, 22
Hepatitis C virus. See also
        Immune system; Liver
    blood, spread by infected, 2, 5–6
    botanical medicines for (See
        Botanical medicines for HCV
        and liver; Botanical support
        for immune system)
    conventional treatment, 3
    description of, 4–6
    as emerging virus, 102, 108
    as epidemic, 1
    family tree of, 11–13, 12
    herbal healing of, 22
    incubation period, 2–3
    infection and disease from, 2–3,
        8–9, 11
    inside view of, 9–11
    major strains, 12–13
    nutritional supplements for (See
        Nutritional supplements for
        HCV)
    population infected by, 2–3
    protocols for (See Protocols,
        HCV)
    related diseases, 21–22
    symptoms of, 2
    tests for, 111–113

Hepatitis D, E, and G, 10
**Hepatitis Soup,** 95
*Herbal Medicine, Healing &*
*Cancer,* 100
Herbal medicines, making/using,
113–119
  alcohol extractions, 116
  children's dosages, 118
  decoctions, 115
  glycerites and honeys, 118–119
  infusions, 114–115
  powders/capsules, 117–118
  tinctures, 116–117
  water extractions, 114
  whole herbs, consuming,
  117–118
Herbs, immune. *See* Botanical
  support for immune system
Herbs, liver. *See* Botanical medi-
  cines for HCV and liver
Herpesvirus saimiri, 106–107
HIV, 9, 102, 108
Honeys, 93, 118–119
Hormones, 21
Hyperglycemia, 20
*Hypericum perfoliatum,* 100
Hypertension, 21–22
Hypoglycemia, 20

**I**
**Immune-Enhancing Rice,** 60
Immune system
  botanical support for (*See*
  Botanical support for
  immune system)
  liver and, 14–15
Indigestion, 100
Infusions, 53, 72, 114–115

Interferon, 1, 3, 12
Interferon-alpha, 15
Interleukin-2, 15
Irritability, 100
Itching. *See* Skin problems

**J**
Jaundice, 2, 4, 17, 43
Joint pain, 100

**K**
Kupffer cells, 15

**L**
Lactobrev, 82
LDL (low-density lipoprotein), 20,
  112
*Leonarus cardiaca. See* Motherwort
*Leptandra virginica,* 101
Libido, low, 21, 101
Licorice *(Glycyrrhiza glabra),* **55,**
  63–65, 92, 98
  contraindications, 65
  preparation/dosage, 64–65
*Ligusticum porterii,* 118
Liver, 14–22, *17*
  bile, 17–18
  biopsy, 113
  botanical medicines for (*See*
  Botanical medicines for HCV
  and liver)
  cancer, 100
  carbohydrate conversion by, 19
  cirrhosis, 2, 21–22, 100
  cycles, effect of HCV on, 18–21
  description of, 16
  diet for (*See* Diet)
  fat breakdown by, 20

Liver (continued)
    filtering process, 16–17
    hormones and enzymes, 20
    immune system and, 14–15
    protein breakdown by, 19
    regeneration, 16
    stabbing pains in region of, 2, 101
Low-fat cleansing diet, 89–95
Lymphoid aggregates, 2

**M**

Macrophages, 14–15
Maple syrup, 93
Marburg virus, 102
Massage, 96, 98, 99, 100, 101
Measles virus, 107
Meat, 19, 92–93, 101
Memory problems, 2
Menstrual disorders, 21, 100
Mental fatigue, 101
Menu, recommended, 93
Milk thistle *(Silybum marianum)*,
    **24,** 37–40
    contraindications, 40
    preparation/dosage, 40
    seeds, 39
    use of, 38–40, 94, 97–101
Mood swings, 2, 21, 100
Motherwort *(Leonarus cardiaca),*
    99, 100, 101
Mullein ( *Verbascum* spp.), 100
Mushrooms, reishi. *See* Reishi
    *(Ganoderma lucidum)*

**N**

N-acetylcysteine (NAC), **77,** 78–79,
    98
    contraindications, 79
    dosage, 79
Nausea, 4, 20, 90, 100
Neck, swelling around, 101
Nettles *(Urtica dioca),* 101
Numbness in extremities, 101
Nutritional supplements for HCV,
    76–82
    alpha-lipoic acid, **77,** 76–78
    B vitamin complex, **77,** 80, 98
    C vitamin, **77,** 80, 98
    E vitamin, **77,** 81–82, 98
    in hepatitis protocols, 98
    lactobrev, 82
    N-acetylcysteine, **77,** 78–79
    selenium, **77,** 79
    zinc, 82

**O**

Oils, 89, 90, 91
*Oplopanax horridum,* 99
Osha root *(Ligusticum porterii),*
    118

**P**

*Paeonia albiflora,* 53
*Paeonia moutan,* 53
*Paeonia rubra,* 52
Pain medications, use of, 84
Panax (or Asian) ginseng *(Panax
    ginseng),* **55,** 65–67, 98, 99,
    100, 101
    contraindications, 67
    preparation/dosage, 67
*Panax pseudoginseng,* var. *notogin-
    seng,* var. *japonicus. See*
    Tienchi ginseng
Pasque flower *(Anemone pusitilla),*
    100

PCR test, 10, 113
Peaches *(Prunus persica),* 90
*Pedicularis* spp., 101
Pestiviruses, 11
*Peumus boldus. See* Boldo
Phyllanthus *(Phyllanthus niruri, P. amarus, P. emblica),* **24,** 40–43
   contraindications, 43
   preparation/dosage, 43
   uses of, 41–43, 97, 98, 101
Picrorhiza *(Picrohiza kurroa),* **24,** 43–45
   contraindications, 45
   preparation/dosage, 45
   uses of, 44–45, 97, 100
Polymerase chain reaction (PCR) test, 10, 113
*Polyporus umbellatus,* 52
*Poria cocos,* 53
Portal hypertension, 21–22
Powders, 117–118
   astralagus, 59
   bupleurum, 31
   burdock, 33
   chlorella, 87
   codonopsis, 62
   dandelion, 37
   licorice, 65
   milk thistle, 40
   panax ginseng, 67
   phyllanthus, 43
   picrorhiza, 45
   reishi, 48
   schizandra, 71
   Siberian ginseng, 72
   spirulina, 89
   turmeric, 51

Protein
   breakdown by liver, 19
   in diet, 89, 92–93
Protocols, HCV, 96–101
   Option 1, 97–98
   Option 2, 98–99
   parts of, 96–97
   premixed formula, 98–99
   specific symptoms, herbs for, 99–101
*Prunus persica,* 90
*Pueraria lobata,* 53
Puffy face, 99

**R**

Raspberry leaf *(Rubus idaeus),* 100
Recipes, 51, 59, 93–95, 115, 117
Red clover *(Trifolium pratense),* 101
Red root *(Ceanothus* spp.), **55,** 67–69, 98, 101
   contraindications, 69
   preparation/dosage, 68–69
*Rehmannia glutinosa,* 53
Reishi *(Ganoderma lucidum),* **24,** 46–48
   contraindications, 48
   preparation/dosage, 48
   recipes, 95, 115
   uses of, 486–47, 97, 99–101
**Reishi Syrup Decoction,** 115
*Rheum officinale,* 52, 90–91
Rhubarb *(Rheum officinale),* 52, 90–91
Ribivarin, 3, 12
RNA, 7–10
*Rubus idaeus,* 100
*Rubus villosus,* 100

## S

Salad dressing, 91
Salt, 90, 91
*Salvia miltiorrhiza*, 53
Schizandra *(Schisandra chinensis)*,
    **55**, 69–71, 98, 99, 100
  contraindications, 71
  preparation/dosage, 71
*Scutellaria baicalensis. See* Baical
    skullcap
Seasonal affective disorder, 100
Seasonings, 91
*Sedum sarmentosum*, 52
Selenium, 79–80
Shellfish, 4
Siberian ginseng *(Eleutherococcus
    senticosus)*, **55**, 71–73, 98–101
  contraindications, 73
  preparation/dosage, 72
*Silybum marianum. See* Milk
    thistle
Skin problems, 2, 17, 101
Sleep, need for, 100, 101
Sleep disorders, 18–19, 92, 101
Smallpox, 107
*Smilax china*, 53
*Solanum nigrum*, 53
Spirulina *(Spirulina platensis)*,
    88–89, 93, 99
  contraindications, 89
  preparation/dosage, 89
  recipes, 95
St.-John's-wort *(Hypericum perfo-
    liatum)*, 100
Steatosis, 2, 20
Sweets, 93
Swelling in armpits, groin, neck,
    101

Symbiogenesis, 103–104
  aggressive symbiosis, 106–108
  viral jumping, 105–106
*Symphytum officinale*, 52

## T

*Tamarix gallica*, 53
*Taraxacum officinale. See*
    Dandelion
Tea, 92, 99. *See also* Green tea
    *(Camellia sinensis)*
  baical skullcap, 26
  bladderwrack, 85
  boldo, 28
  boneset, 61
  bupleurum, 31
  burdock, 33
  dandelion, 36
  decaffeinating, 88
  licorice, 65
  phyllanthus, 43
  red root, 69
  Siberian ginseng, 72
*Terminalia arjuna*, 53
Tests
  hepatitis C virus, 111–113
  hepatitis G virus, 10
Tienchi ginseng *(Panax pseudogin-
    seng,* var. *notoginseng,* var.
    *japonicus)*, **55**, 73–75, 97, 98, 99
Tinctures, 116–117
  astralagus, 58
  bladderwrack, 85
  boldo, 28
  boneset, 61
  burdock, 33
  *Carduus nutans*, 52
  dandelion, 36

licorice, 64
milk thistle, 40
panax ginseng, 67
picrorhiza, 45
red root, 68
reishi, 48
schizandra, 71
Siberian ginseng, 72
tienchi ginseng, 75
turmeric, 51
*Trifolium pratense,* 101
T (thymus) cells, 15
Turmeric *(Curcuma longa),* **24,**
   48–51
contraindications, 51
preparation/dosage, 51
recipes, 51, 95
uses of, 49–50, 91, 97, 98, 100
**Turmeric Paste,** 51

**U**
Urination, frequent, 100
*Urtica dioca,* 101

**V**
Vaccinations, 4, 6
Vegetables, 90–91, 94, 98, 100
*Verbascum* spp., 100
*Vigna sinensis,* 53
Viruses
   aggressive symbiosis, 106–108
   classifications of, 7–8

discovery of, 104
DNA and, 7–10, 104–105, 107
emerging, 102–110
function of, 103–104
hepatitis A, 4, 11
hepatitis B, 6
hepatitis C (*See* Hepatitis C virus)
hepatitis D, E, and G, 10
how they infect, 2–3, 8–9, 11
human culture, effect of, 109–110
viral jumping, 105–106
viral swarm, 10
Vitamin B complex, 80, 98
Vitamin C, 80–81, 98
Vitamin E, 81–82, 98
Vitex *(Vitex agnus-castus),* 100

**W**
Water, 89, 91
Water extractions, 114
Weakness, 100
West Nile virus, 11, 102
*Withania somnifera. See*
   Ashwagandha
Wood betony (*Pedicularis* spp.), 101

**Y**
Yance, Donald, 100

**Z**
Zinc, 82, 98

# OTHER BOOKS IN THE STOREY MEDICINAL HERB GUIDE SERIES

*ADHD Alternatives,* by Aviva Romm and Tracy Romm. 160 pages. Paperback. ISBN 1-58017-248-2.

*Healthy Bones and Joints,* by David Hoffmann. 128 pages. Paperback. ISBN 1-58017-253-9.

*Herbal Antibiotics,* by Stephen Harrod Buhner. 144 pages. Paperback. ISBN 1-58017-148-6.

*Herbal Remedies for Children's Health,* by Rosemary Gladstar. 80 pages. Paperback. ISBN 1-58017-153-2.

*Herbal Remedies for Men's Health,* by Rosemary Gladstar. 96 pages. Paperback. ISBN 1-58017-151-6.

*The Herbal Home Remedy Book,* by Joyce E. Wardwell. 176 pages. Paperback. ISBN 1-58017-016-1.

*Herbs for the Home Medicine Chest,* by Rosemary Gladstar. 96 pages. Paperback. ISBN 1-58017-156-7.

*Rosemary Gladstar's Family Herbal,* by Rosemary Gladstar. 408 pages. Paperback. ISBN 1-58017-425-6.

*Saw Palmetto for Men & Women,* by David Winston. 128 pages. Paperback. ISBN 1-58017-206-7.

*These and other books from Storey Publishing are available wherever quality books are sold or by calling 1-800-441-5700.*
*Visit us at www.storey.com.*